DIALYSIS 2121

Sujata Kohli

Invincible Publishers

First published in India in 2018

ISBN: 978-93-87328-32-7

Invincible Publishers

G-120, Sushant Lok III, Sector 57, Gurgaon-122002

Registered Address: Opposite Kasturba Ashram, Radaur, Haryana - 135133

I dedicate my book in the fond memory of my mother and to the patients who are in misery to run from pillar to post.

ACKNOWLEDGEMENT

Towards achieving my object, in the form of this humble attempt of a book, I have been encouraged through only by my colleague and friend Sh. Narender Kumar, Ld Additional Sessions Judge, Delhi, and also who was there whenever I had lost …the zest......to go on, being over burdened with the professional commitments, at those moments, it is he who used to encourage and motivate me to complete the same, reminding me about my main object behind this book.

Further, I have to acknowledge all my gratitude to Dr. prof B.M. Hegde who was magnanimous enough to grant permission to me, to include his esteemed articles in this book, to emphasise the point I tried to make, but would not have been able to make, without the aid of such articles, authored by a senior medical professional.

Infact, Dr. Prof B.M. Hegde can be said to have given me the honour to include such articles herein, for which I am deeply indebted.

Contents

RECALL ON THE MOUNTAIN ROAD

Wipers moving fast, it was raining cats and dogs; the winding road, mountains faded into the thick clouds, roaring winds, screeching of the brakes, the slippery road and the echoes take me back somewhere into my childhood…………" Barnala, Bansot, Ameel………Kahan ho tum………..Barnala, Bansot……………."

The winds are roaring, lightening in the sky, the steep slopes keep me going cautiously, but the rain goes on incessantly……."water……….water……….Paani Do……..". The nurse comes and wipes the dry parched lips with wet cotton wool and says, "Please, have water." Tears blind my vision. Rain mingles with my tears. So much water around………..not a drop for her. The smiling angelic face brightening up at the prospect of water. And then the disappointment…………..the torture of being deprived of even one drop

A sudden sharp turn and a huge tree in the middle of the road and then the collision …………..lights in the ICU are very dim. I have people whispering around me ……………..why she was driving in the rain without the wipers on . Little could they see what

I saw behind the rain, was the figure of that smiling angelic face proceeding towards me asking for water……just one drop……..but denied.

UPROOTED FROM THE LAP

My first day at school comes to me as a flash of light. The two piggie tails perched on the top of each corner of my head…new pink colour check frock with belt tied prim, my new black strap shoes…..but all these could not console me at all when the butter colour ambassador driven by daddy ,carrying me and 'Billy', came to a halt before the over bearing and the formidable building with red bricks, grey colour window panes displaying the big board 'LADY IRWIN GIRLS' JUNIOR SCHOOL'…….

I continued with my incessant tantrums. The feeling of being uprooted from the mother's warm lap, out into the cold and damp world. My first taste of the outer world, out of the shelter of my mother's world was almost unacceptable…but then came my 'second mother' and took over charge. She was my saviour and ultimately was my consolation when she took me to her own class in the Vth standard. I was the apple of the eye of all concerned.

But prior to this I had to go through a miserable time when I landed up in another class room, and the concerned teacher, came upto me, caught hold of my arm, twisting and pulling it, she brought me out and I cannot forget how small I felt and how all this added to my agony of the separation from my 'Billy'

Please forgive me Billy…….

Atlast my second mother took good care of me and ultimately my first and worst day at school was over.

Steaming hot paranthas, the aroma from the kitchen window, I rushed inside leaving my friends and the game in the middle..my cute fat Billy was busy as ever….

I remember the afternoon when after finishing school, I was dropped at the bus stop, but from the bus stop till home I got drenched completely in the rain, pouring cats and dogs. My paternal aunt had arrived for a visit. Special kinds of food were being prepared. My Billy got worried seeing me all drenched. She put me on the nearby stool, changed my wet clothes and made me warm and cozy, brought me and made me take a glass of warm milk…that angel was just around when I needed her most.

THE PAPER BOATS IN THE RAIN

The house was brimming with lot of events going on……………on so lively………..

The three sided corner flat with a garden on each side, the front garden facing the old Fort, the back garden facing the neighbours House No.5…the side garden was full of home grown carrots, onions, radish, potato and what not….Three mango trees in the front garden, a cactus plant in a corner, a Gulmohar in the right corner…the Cana plants with the red flowers, the rose beds…was it my nice cute home or heaven? The rains would come leashing, all the trees, plants, flowers braving the strong winds, all turning a deep beautiful green….Me, Ajay and other friends would make those paper boats.

Shade of that plum tree in the back garden, was my study room, where she would teach me daily…Monday…Social sciences…Tuesday..English…skip one day of studies, and I had it. She would slap me hard. No way to avoid studies, come rain, or come storm. My 'Billy' would not budge.

Deepawali Fair at the junior school meant for Ist-Vth standard children; all kids were asked to bring toys for the stalls. Like all parents, my mother had also come, but along with one lady, working in our house, but who was more like our family member. My class teacher objected through me there and then. However, I never passed it on to my sweet mom, as I could never tolerate anything, which would belittle her…my cute fat mom.

Too much stomach pain. This small naughty child had to be treated urgently. Doctor was rushed in…medicines, hot water…hot oil…my Billy was on her toes…she did not sleep the whole night.

I would always admire her, when she got ready to go out, she was all grace personified. The fair transparent complexion, untouched skin, no blemishes, no make over…simple home made milk cream, warm water, and she was done…the midsize red bindi…the white saree with the red border. She was my ideal… I kept strolling after and around her, playing with the 'pallu' end. I would always ask her to bring some toy or other…the latest fancy…`the bride and the groom', the `dinner set', the `bedroom drawing room set'…the list was never ending. I would accompany her wherever she went, whether to friends house or to my grandmother's house.

My grandmother always teased my mother for carrying me everywhere as I was the youngest and perhaps the pet.

THE HOUSE IN THE MOUNTAINS

Here comes the summer vacation approaching, hearts full of excitement, me and my second mother Anjali, doing things together, bathing in the rain, dancing, counting our oncoming joyful events like elder brother coming home from Engineering College at Jamalpur, eldest sister coming from MAMC Hostel, their friends also accompanying them, holidays, movies and above all, the packing for the hill station..

"Mommy please start packing"..our plans for the journey…Shimla…Nainital. Mother's phone call to the stores for provisions…the Cane trunk would be taken off the highest shelf..the `hold alls'.

She would take all of us, the children alone…Daddy would come to see us off at the Ajmeri Gate Bus Stand, (then ISBT Bus stand), or at New Delhi Railway Station…It was Daddy's option not to go leaving behind his patients. He was deeply and dedicatedly into homoepathic practice…So, she, my mother would brave it all. The search for the hotel rooms which provided cooking facilities..Uphill..downhill..I remember the spirit.

"Children, do not worry. God helps those who help themselves…I am hopeful and confident…Why then you children are not?"

The best room found with the right location. It used to be a suite..two bedroom, kitchen, path. Now she would make tea for all of us and then the delicious food.

A brown colour centipede on the sofa…we all screamed, but she, the brave heart, picked it up with a metal `chimta'. She was able to get rid of the fast moving centipede.

Soon hot tea would be brewing. We all huddled up in the blankets my mother would be preparing something milk or warm for us to eat.

THE YELLOW CRAZE

I was really fond of that yellow 'Romper' with 2 cats patch work. So fond, that almost attached, and almost obsessed. I would reject all other dresses, cute pretty tunics, party……but simply find out the 'Romper' from the cupboard, and wear it.

It started getting noticed. Mother kept telling, but I would not listen. Lots of fears were put in my mind if I wore the same 'Romper' over and over again. I would not budge.

Finally, my elder brother (fondly referred by me as 'Papa ji' there being huge age gap, I looked upon him as a father figure who had been also present at home from his hostel at Jamalpur, where he was studying engineering) threw it away!

I became shocked and was unsonsolable, when 'Papaji' simply lifted that 'Romper' and threw it onto the top of a large Mango tree in the garden.

Crying, howling it was just unbelievable for me. The warm cozy lap of my mother also could not put me at rest.

Ultimately, I convinced my mom to tell the gardener to bring it down for me. Weeping still, my nose running; still secretly happy; but before the secret could be out, my brother came snatched the 'romper' and threw it into a 'nallah' far off; and thus I lost it forever. I slept crying, weeping; in the lap of my mommy, my 'Billy'. That was my world.

GRACE PERSONIFIED

I would continuously play with the pallu corner of her saree, admire her when she would be sitting before the dressing table; so simple and so beautiful.

Homemade pure milk cream was her face wash. Washed cleaned, glowing, she would put a maroon red colour large 'bindi' and she was done. The pure silk saree, white base with a Red border, the epitome of grace, sobriety, glow and purity of the heart; she would walk as my ideal; holding my hand, taking me along wherever to go; and I would never think of staying behind ever. I was only her shadow, meant to follow her wherever....

Both parents had to go to Banaras, and to Jamalpur in connection with studies of my brother 'Papaji' (He being the eldest I being only a kind used to address him as papa ji) and also to get darshan of some disciple of Swami Yoganandji as my father was also a devotee. I was not allowed to accompany, mainly for my schools being open, and I was not allowed to take leave.

Miserable, I finally was given the promise of a new play kitchen set. It was a short trip by air and they both returned. My happiness knew no bounds. My

Billy was there. My 'kitchen set' was there. It was a golden sunny day in the winters. I would not just stop playing, joy brimming in my little heart with the presence of my mother in the kitchen; cooking nice delicious gajar halwa, the flavour drawing me close, running around here and there like a bee, not being able to wait for it to be done.

EVENINGS AT NAINITAL

About 4 p.m, it is time for going out to the Mall Road. My mommy is tied after the house work, and not wanting to go. But the elder sisters/brother would get bored and as such they all are to go. I am suffering from stomach ache. Mommy convinced me to stay back with 'Mama'. She got that pair of 'bride and bridegroom' for me. I would not seize to get them married to each other every day, mimicking the pandit's mantras.

We would be rendered short of the budget planned for the trip. One time meal i.e. lunch used to be prepared at the accommodation hired by us and dinner would be outdoors. One or two days used to be reserved for boating; one day at Chaat house, with two dishes to each of us; and then one day for shopping; one item to each of us. My mommy would bear the worry, the tension all by herself. She would then be accompanied by the elder children to make a phone call from a PCO to Daddy, who would arrange and send the deficient amount.

THE KARM YOGI

She saw some days very tough. An 'Aryasamajist', she did not believe in idol worship, in gurus etc. and no blind follower of any rituals. Her motto in life was 'work is worship' and 'God helps those who help themselves'. She liked to sing bhajans on 'harmonium' which she played extremely well and naturally. I would also accompany her to the kirtans held in different houses in the colony, every Tuesday.

My grandmother 'Naani' would often remark to her "Vimla why do you always carry her with you? Does she not leave you alone for a minute even? She won't let us talk/chit-chat, undisturbed'. It is the elder children who were the favourites of my 'Naani'. Anyhow, I would not care and nor would my Billy, who would just laugh it off, chiding my grandmother, for saying this for me, in my presence. I would continue playing in that *gali* of South Extn. Block B with the children around. By 5, it would be time to return home. My 'Nana' would give some money to her and me both would return home.

MY MENTOR

'Elephant?-Elephant. This is the topic I have to write about, if I wished to be selected for further study after IIIrd class, in English medium. Mommy, what do I write? Tell me…..And lo ! The language, the natural flow and the foundation laid by her….all led to not only my selection but a special word of praise from my teacher.

I as always in a hurry to complete my tests at school. I would do very well but always stood 2nd in rank but never Ist. She always would hold her head in exasperation, the moment I would reveal the answer of the last question, always wrongly, and only out of omission/carelessness. My teachers would always write remarks on my report…..intelligent, hardworking but 'careless'. And I would just laugh it off.

Mommy would spend hours teaching me each evening. During annuals or half yearlies she would continue till 2 A.M., the night; would then sprinkle water on my sleepy eyes. Then again she would get up at 5 a.m. in the morning, to cook for me to take to school. "Mommy, please take one round of the kitchen. I'll get up…just one more round…"

She would often lightly tell others… "this youngest daughter of mine really troubles me so much….she makes me run here and there all the time".

THE SIZZLING FOOD

There was this cricket match on, 5 day match between India and Australia. My eldest brother and sister were home on vacation from their hostels; Their friends from around…all about 10 or 15 gathered in the drawing room, all glued to the T.V. My poor 'Billy' preparing aaloo paranthas for each one …on or on…her legs swollen, but happily and joyously cooking endlessly.

Returning from India Gate after a morning walk, all of us would be taking bath and Mommy would be busy blending the curd with the old manual churning rod, to prepare 'Lassi'.

THE SLAP AT THE LAKE

We had reached Nainital. Luggage was taken off from the roof of the bus, and when it was discovered that my mother's suitcase had been lost/dropped/fallen on the way. My 'Mama' (later on found by me to be my brother by blood, having given away in adoption by my mother to her own mother) was showing the beauty of the hills and the lake surrounded by them…and a thud of a resounding slap on his face…and by whom? My mommy had slapped him hard. I did not like and sympathized with my 'Mama'.

Today, I cry, remembering my mother, who had lost most of her expensive valuable sarees, pashmina shawls, jewelry; on that trip. In fact, she had to buy two sarees, and had to spend the entire trip on those clothes. She had specifically asked 'Mama' to keep checking the luggage on the roof when others had checked, but he had taken it lightly and my poor mother's most favorite belongings were lost.

However, apart from that slap I never saw her even frown or crib on any other day of the entire twenty or twenty five days trip. Our trips used to be long stays in rented cottages, or portions thereof or rented rooms equipped with kitchen.

All 12 bananas had disappeared. And who had eaten them but me. I had concealed myself under the table and ate each, one by one. She did not know whether to get angry, or to laugh, at seeing my mouth full.

Life kept on like a smooth sail boat. Soft, straight, slightly bending-curving. The self breeze the rainy days, the house made from two upright beds, with the tarpaulin as a roof, me or my friends playing the 'Ghar Ghar', our favourite game…raining cats and dogs, the simmering tea, the pakoras prepared with her loving hands, were brought by me to that tarpauline house, to make the house real.

….the cold winter misty evenings, the long walks with Daddy full Raj Path, Rashtrapati Bhawan, eating 'Moongphali' (peanuts), pockets full, me returned home to see her crying, requesting my daddy to try for transfer of my brother, her only son to Delhi.

TRIP TO ADRA - THE HURT

Eldest sister, eldest brother got married off on alternte days. I had now been promoted to Vth standard. Happy and joyous with the ongoing celebrations, freedom from studies….life was running these days. I was on cloud nine. The favourite of my eldest brother and eldest sister, the baby of the house…these days I was not the shadow of my mother…she was too…busy…and I was too…busy playing whole day.

Me and my elder sister known as my 2nd mother were traveling by train to go to Adra, near Aasansol in West Bengal, to visit 'Papaji'…Train had taken a change of line somewhere near Agra. Taj was visible. Mommy was sleeping. We were in the ladies compartment. Suddenly, I observed this burka clad lady, sitting near my Mommy, indulging in bad habits, like 'digging' and then sticking the dirt nearby….

No…I could not tolerate…just got up woke my mommy up and I told her to watch and be alert. My sweet innocent mother woke up puzzled thinking she was at home cooking…then remembering…smiling at me.. happy at the thought of visiting her dear son, the apple of her eye. She looked at that woman, stared at her, indirectly telling her to stop in her activity…Thank God she desisted…

Welcome by 'Papaji' at Adra was just great. We were givn the ride in the 'Saloon' meant for very senior Railway Officers like the Dy. CME..It was thrilling, this bunglow, the sprawling lawns, almost forest, litee, the swing…the cottage like look all just too good.

Yet the hurt in the eyes of my mother, caused by the ill behaviour of his wife, could not be concealed from my watchful eyes. I was always the little body guard of my mother…no one dare hurt her…

Days, into weeks, weeks into months and months into years passed. She would be just busy in kitchen, one thing or another. Her day would start at 5 in the morning, and would not close until 12 in the mid night. Her ankles would get swollen, but on and on, she would continue.

THE FOREIGN LAND

On account of family exigency my Billy had to go to the United States all by herself. Scared and nervous she was but that did not deter the bold lady. She reached there by herself, managed and succeeded in her purpose. Though she suffered much and so did father who joined her later in the U.S. How they both wept on their return that July morning. I shall never forget…

Life went on as usual. My mother was my closest friend, companion, to play Ludo indoors while it was raining outside, taking the nice warm cup of coffee together in the early mornings of the monsoon season, to lie down and laze around on the terrace, in the winter afternoons, to drive around in my Omni on the long drives, away from the hub of the city, to accompany me to my Himachal trips after every two three months..

THE NYLON TENT PROJECT AND THE BUBBLE

One winter afternoon, the plans had been made for a tent on the terrace for both of us, to enjoy camping life style, as and when we felt like; but before it could materialize and take shape, she was discouraged and dissuaded by some family member regarding some hazards involved and it was shelved.

The next 'project' was for construction of a room on the terrace, meant for being enjoyed during rain, where tea and snacks could be prepared and which would give us a good view all around, with French windows on all three sides. The second project actually took shape…and we all in the family, saw many a good times, in that room, which gave the look of a tourist bungalow in some hill place.

While on a long journey to a far off place, with myself driving and my Billy sitting beside me, she would request, then demand and then insist for fruity, kurkure both of which were barred for her by the doctors. Upon the demand being met, she would laugh, her eyes twinkling, and taking each sip and bite ,she would relish, and then condemn the doctors as being absolutely un knowledgeable about the heart, soul and mind of a person.

She was cheerful person by nature. Never the one to complain or to harbor grievances. Each trip to the mountains would simply exhilarate her so much. She would be most enthusiastic.

I hardly ever saw her down with any ailment, not even as much as a fever, but whatever minor problem would be there, she would minimize it even further. Her principle was really a cure by natural process. No `mycins' for her. Either it was a 'tulsi tea' or a herbal preparation called 'joshanda'.

Upon her being afflicted with some rashes on her feet, all that she treated it with, was an oil massage with mustard oil. Insistence by eldest sister upon her to take anti biotiques failed. And what more! Within a few days of repeated process, her both feet were just as fine as ever. Then again she would simply laugh and rebuke all medical sciences.

MY SAVIOUR

It was the Navmi puja .I was distributing Prasad. Silently, unknowingly, the flames of the 'jyot' had caught up with my chlothes. By the time I realized, a substantial portion of the top 'kurti' worn by me had been caught into flames. Not able to even think what I should do to escape, and with only a few kids around ,none to help me, God appeared silently in the form of my angelic Mother, just from nowhere. Our house being on a longish plot, the rooms had been constructed on both sides of a long running gallery, right from one end to the other. I had been on the extreme west of the house in the pooja room, while she had been sitting in the extreme east part of the house being the drawing room, and in her daily routine Mother would not have come all that far at that time of the day. It was nothing but her intuition. She just waved and literally put off the flames by her hands, not hesitating even and for a moment. That is Mother. That is God.

TRIP TO MASROOR - MY GUILT

In the approaching winter months I had somehow managed to sneak out a trip for myself to my second home i.e. Dharamshala. And of course my partner could not stay behind. She and me moved on by the Himachal roadways bus and when in the town we were commuting by taxi mostly.

I persuaded her to accompany me to the 'Masroor' temple which was a very ancient temple known for its unique monolithique architecture, as the entire structure had been carved out of a single rock. The route was beautiful winding, hairpin like bends surrounded by greenery all around. I was lost in my own world, and kept nudging at her for a response to the scene spread around. That poor sacrificing soul kept responding, albeit a little feebly, but I failed to notice. Brimming with my enthusiasm, I helped her alight from the taxi, which also happened to be a Maruti Omni. With my help and some assistance from the driver, she managed to cross that rocky and rough patch. It was when I held her small soft hand, that to my utter dismay and a feeling of shame, that I found that my mother was suffering from a very high fever. Full of guilt, having been lost in my own world, I had failed to take note of the agony my mother must have been going through, all this while when she kept giving responses to my silly chatter at the appropriate points and sharing my small joys and surprises.

I immediately made her sit on a railing and brought tea for her along with some biscuits to go. But poor thing, she was suffering too much. I insisted we go back immediately but the brave and spirited person that she was, she was determined that I go around the whole temple, see it and only thereafter we would return. My natural interest and curiosity about that temple got the better of me and I got mesmerized, seeing that unique monolithic structure, and once again could not hide my excitement. Once again I set out to describe the interiors to her, forgetting about her condition. What could I do when she kept smiling and looking happy at my joy.

We returned in the late afternoon and on way back, showing her to a local doctor. On return to Delhi that she was suffering from a very painful skin condition called 'herpes'. Honestly I got scared, but how my mother spent that period just peacefully without any complaints, was exemplary.

THE ROAD TO DHARAMSHALA LOST

It was one of those months when winter starts to set in, with the haze, smog, fog pollution all mixed, the hour when the sun rays are sans their warmth, the sun assumes a pinkish shade, villagers are starting to return to the warmth of their small cozy homes, the cyclists in a row, the birds flying in their flocks to their nests, the chill slowly setting in, me and my mother also quite wrapped up in our Van still too far from our destination, having taken some wrong route. By that moment, we were chasing time and had barely managed to reach till kiratpur only. I kept telling her to lie down and catch up with some sleep, as we had a long way to go. Neither she agreed to lie down, nor to take dinner, and was adamant that she would have it at the destination only, and not before. I gave up just irritatedly, but concealing my smile, I kept driving.

The race against time was now over and we continued our journey at a steady pace through the dark forests and spread out fields, the head lights piercing the surroundings showing safely closed houses, people having already retired for the night, after the hard day's work. My twelve hour drive, which had converted into a sixteen hour one, was nowhere near its end. We both made best of the worst, with her constant encouraging remarks, and the next moment her probing question “how far now?”

Feeling very bad for her, I kept trying that she would take dinner somewhere, but in vain. Crossing various bridges, hair pin bends, the steep ascents, finally I could see the shimmering lights of the town at last. Feeling encouraged, I increased the speed, and after half an hour or so, when the entire town was also asleep, my small Van entered the town of Dharamshala. At that unearthly hour, we could not hope for any dinner, and my poor Billy had to make do with just a glass of milk, a banana and some Uncle Chips. Receiving my looks of “Look I told you so” and scolding, she lapped up the food items, whatever were available, covering up her disappointment, by a smile. She was really hungry and infact we both were. However awaiting the morning, we both ended up fast asleep.

SUNSETS IN THE WINTER

Winter was setting in. My 'Billy' was preparing, and there she goes, in that dugduggi of a cycle rickshaw, tumbling all the way, to the 'razaiwala'. She was further on her shopping trip, some new and attractive crockery, some other household goods; and on her way back, there would be a treat of a large glass of juice for all concerned, including the rickshaw puller. All including the shopkeeper would be her 'son'.

THE AFTERNOON WALKS TO SANJOULI SHIMLA

Afternoon walks upto sanjouli tunnel, would bring out the instant story from her about the good old days, her only son, and how she, my dad and they all used to walk up to miles and miles even up till Tara Devi. Some of our group would be laughing, some would be irritated by the repetitive stories, but I just used to look at her with awe, admiring her throughout, cherishing and absorbing each and every word uttered from her lips, as if somewhere deep down, even as a child, I knew that this voice would not be there forever. Somewhere along the way, I would drown into the past narrated by her, almost re-living it myself, though I had not seen it.

The Ridge road, the old English Church, stand witness to those moments when she would crave for an ice-cream and after a lot of beseeching and almost begging, she would be thrilled to get it. How she would be busy for sometimes to come, totally engrossed in the ice cream, not a care in the world. Her twinkling bright eyes, would become brighter with even the thought of an ice-cream or a chocolate.

The house in Tooti Kandi, the verandah therein, all used to be huddle up in blankets, at a far off distance, we could see the ever continuing fires in the forests. Mom would be preparing hot and sizzling food, ready to serve us all the time.

Whether it was the question of walking up to Jhaku Temple, or whether it was China Peak or Vaishno Devi Shrine, she would always pick up the courage, the determination, just for the sake of accompanying me, and fulfilling my wish and desire, as she herself did not believe in rituals etc. Be it a centipede or a Scorpio, or any such creepy creature, she would not be behind to deal with it, come what may. Be it a thunder storm or any other calamity, she would not be the one to be deterred. Like a pillar of courage and boldness, she was all the time around us, and I felt so nurtured all the time in my cocoon of security and warm.

It was a trip in Darjeeling, Sikkim etc, while in Sikkim, on a tiff with my niece and nephew and cousins, I was left alone and isolated. But she always understood and saw everything without my needing to tell her.

RECOVERY AT NAINITAL

Once after recovering from a long illness, I persisted in my wish to go to Nainital. She had agreed earlier, but may be in a casual manner, not rarely expecting that I would continue seriously with my intentions. Once I continued to press, poor thing, she budged in.

Arrangements were supposed to be made by Dad through a friend of his but it is only the 'Billy' and myself who were going alone by bus. It was the October month and in those days, it used to be chilly enough in that time of the year also.

Somewhere along the Kumau forests belt, the bus broke down. I still cannot forget how me and 'Billy' passed our time chatting.

We were both sitting near the tyre which was lying on the road and we had much to discuss, some in eagerness to reach the destination, and some in anxiety about as to what kind of arrangement would be there for our stay and what time we are going to reach Nainital.

It was quite late, around 9:00 PM that our bus reached the banks of the lake towards Tallital side. It was quite chilly as the wind was blowing. Me and

'Billy' took a rickshaw to the other end of the lake road.

From there, little bit could be imagined what lay in store for us. Miles and miles of steep climbing and the house was nowhere to be seen. I felt worried for Mom and very guilty, that I had brought her due to my stubbornness, poor thing, she kept walking and walking, on and on, taking rest in between, but not once did she blame me, on the contrary it was she who was cheering up me and encouraging me to go on. Once at the house, we both were in for a shock and what more than that, it was absolutely suffocating and unthinkable for us to spend even a night there. All windows and doors closed tight, not a whiff of fresh air to be felt, the silence itself killing both of us. I whispered in her ears, that first thing in the morning, I would go and look for an independent accommodation. She immediately agreed as ever.

Low on the budget, but I was lucky and managed to find a reasonably good, comfortable and well ventilated room having a good view of the lake, I immediately paid the advance and rushed back to fetch my 'Billy', lest she be persuaded by the host, to continue to stay there.

Once we were out on to the road, it was like a breath of fresh air and freedom, and we both were joyful. Sun was shining and causing shimmer in the lake, and unforgettable scenes from in between the tall trees along the road. The multi-coloured beautiful yachts dotting the lake, and then came my next demand, that I want to go for boating. She assured me that if the budget permits towards the end, on the last day, we can go boating once. Satisfied, I held to her hand, looking up to her as if wanting another assurance. She kept smiling. The cycle rickshaw tugged on…

THE SHARING

The first ever interaction between us when she told me exclusively, the interest story about the events that led to her own marriage, was unique. We both were intended to go to Bhimtal that day, but we had missed the bus and also she had broken her slippers. Ultimately we have to return to the room as it was late to start for Bhimtal. She did not want to go anywhere locally. As such we both became lazy, and kept huddled in the quilts, looking at the lake and somehow the discussion started and turned towards the extreme past. She talked for hours and I just listened, mesmerized! She bore a yellow saree with a white frill and the long sleeved yellow blouse. I just laughed, not believing that a bride could where a yellow colour saree. But then that was the custom. Now I just imagined how beautiful she must have looked.

Surprisingly next day, when I was still lazy, she was the one very determined to start for Bhimtal, early in the morning and she pulled me along. Once there, we both had the promise boat ride in the deep waters of Bhimtal, and went up to the island. There was not a joy she spared to give me. The expensive plate of 'Rajma rice', the fancy photograph, she would not deny me anything if possible…….

However, I should have expected and yes, we did go low on the budget and there it hit the hardest. I was told by her to cut down on the dinner menu as we were running out. I felt very small and unconfident, insecure, but then not for long. She managed somehow and assured me it was not all that bad after all.

RED FOR THE GREEN

Transformer had exploded and the bad news, that there would not be any light for another four days. The entire locality was dipped into darkness. My routine duty was to prepare the dinner. While I was still chopping onions in the candle light, feeling bad for me, she suggested, we get food on phone. Thrilled but still in doubt as to whether Dad would like it, even he was magnanimous and immediately I gave the call and the food was there at the gate.

Excited, while I was trying to take out the 'paneer' into the bowl, it would not come out of the polythene packing. Just wondering, I brought the candle close, and in the focused light, what I saw, shocked me. The said 'paneer' finally dropped into the bowl, but it turned out to be not 'paneer' but a chicken or some other non-vegetarian material. Scared to death, mainly of my father, I sneaked to my mother's room and whispered to her about this. I immediately called up to the restaurant.

The exchange was done, but this time no 'paneer' but only 'dal' which was a safe bet. Dad did not come to know about any of this. This was also a secret, only between me and her. Then came the night and we kept chatting into the late hours, we were to sleep outside in the back lawn. Those were the days and that was the kind of Delhi.

JOURNEY TO NARNAUL MY COMPANION IN MY TRIP

There was this case at Narnaul in which I had been engaged as lawyer. I had planned to go by a bus but upon her insistence, to accompany me on the trip, I decided to venture out in my own Omni. A friend of mine was also accompanying us. My mother enjoyed the trip, and was just at our level, and in fact she was a third friend.

I was to leave for Narnaul for the case of my client. And there she goes! Both of us finally after so much arguments, could be seen boarding the roadways bus from Nizzammuddin. Once on the way, while I was listening to my favourite music through my headphone, the curious 'Billy' wanted to feel how it sounded. I put the headphones on her. Chuckling all along, she got into the music, and would not leave the headphones. There was a particular number she laughed and somehow she described it and referred to it in all times to come telling me to play it repeatedly, 'zanjeeren,' that is the name she gave to the song.

The song echoes, while I drive up the hills, try to find her around me, but I cannot. She is not there. But I feel her around. 'Samay' was the other song from 'Rudali', which would make her get lost into the memories. But not for long. She liked to live in the present and to enjoy each moment of life, come what may.

THE DREAMS AND THE ASHES FLOW

The banks of Ganges, the steps, in the distance flow the ashes…… There goes my 'Billy'….. May be I follow along the banks, keep track, so I can even reach, where the river would meet the Bay of Bengal, just so I can go on getting a glimpse of her. That is not to be. Once she is out of sight, I look up to the hills around, the way to Neel Kanth temple, where I took her along in my van and she was almost my helper as she would be there in all my self-driven journeys to far off places. The trip to Rishikesh, to Shimla, Dharmshala, Dalhousie, all pervasive is her presence.

Till three days after, she had left all of us, I was not willing to eat, the fourth day in the morning, she came to me and got up smiling, telling me, that all had given up but not me, and then she asked for tea and toast. I rushed and brought it, thereafter, she held my hand and asked me to accompany her to others. I took her around and back, she was peaceful. The raindrops would often come on the windscreen of my car but there was no rain.

THE PARAGLIDERS OF BIR AND BILLING

There were days when we both would be alone at home, Dad having gone to clinic at South Extension, we both would play Lido.

I was keen to go and learn paragliding, however, I disclosed to her only, that I wanted to watch it. The steep ascent of 19 kms, on the narrow jeepable road was taking us to Billing, near Bir (Himachal Pradesh), but, not once did I see even a sign of any fear on her face, not even she was on the gorge side. She just enjoyed the music, along with me, not once did she discourage me while I was driving. We were up there, and she was left sitting in the van, while I rushed to the paragliders and disappeared from her sight. I had saved a good Rs.2500/- as pocket money to spend on a ride with a paraglider. I was still working out everything, when suddenly a young Tibetan girl came up to me, and told me that my mother was calling me. Exasperated, I returned to the van, and tried to deny my intentions and my attempt. She then beseeched upon me, and made me swear upon her, that I would not indulge in this super-adventure. Left with no choice, after watching some more paragliders enjoying, I just kept my promise, and we both returned.

A BRUSH WITH THE MEDICINES

The 'doctor' in the family would visit from the U.S. and take her for medical check ups. My 'Billy' would always resist, as she had no problem, and being a happy go lucky person, did not like fuss to be made about her. Actually, even I never liked it. I liked to see and know her only as my hail and hearty spirited travel partner. She was not keen to take any medicine even for a fever.

I had returned from court in the evening, and I saw her in the kitchen as usual preparing tea. I felt, she was not looking well, but I could not expect she was suffering from quite high fever and even swelling on feet. I remember today, she had been given a tablet to control urine, by our doctor saab in a very casual manner, ie when she was in the U.S., just so that we would not have to stop on the high ways. Neither I, nor my mother must have realized at that point of time, what this would lead to, one day. Upon seeing her condition, I asked her to consume a tablet of paracitemol but my Billy wouldn't budge. Neither daddy nor anyone else was able to convince her to take medicine, and ultimately I had to call my Mama/brother to manage and to compell her. Her fever was rising by the minute and seeing her swollen feet, I was too scared. Ultimately she was give n a sleep tablet mixed in water and unwittingly she consumed it. She was transferred to the van and taken to Holy Family Hospital.

Within a week she had recovered fully, and was her same self, laughing, chatting, as ever and we both were on to our trips.

She had accompanied me to Rhishi Kesh, and was constantly complaining about restlessness or suffocation. I had become worried but she was not. In the daytime, she would be just normal, but her discomfort was there only in the nights.

THE ROSE - WITHERS

However upon our return from Rhishikesh, it was the republic day and at about 8 p.m., she complained the first time in her life, and she herself told me to take her to the hospital or to a doctor. Being the youngest child, and never having been given any opportunity to take initiative, and to take decisions, here was a major situation before me, and myself being alone, and none to guide me, I was quite nervous, never having seen my mother complaining about her health, my mother herself being the pillar of support for me.

I had not much time to think or to waiver. I simply made her sit in my van and took her to the closest nursing home, which was owned and run by the regular doctor under whose guidance she had been after being detected with diabetes, commonly occurring by advanced age. Upon examining her, doctors recommended me to take he to a bigger hospital with all requisite facilities, as her ECG was showing changes. To be honest, till my interaction with all these events, I was not even aware what it meant. Nor did I realize what was now in store for my 'Billy'.

I got her shifted to a local hospital, feeling too nervous, and just wondering what would be the fate. Things were not managed in the said hospital at a fast pace. On the contrary they were irritatingly slow and leading to much anxiety.

I would seek and expect God to bring improvement and development every half hour or so, thereafter, the hours merged into days, nights, and into more than even a week. Almost ten days had gone by, since her admission to the so called ICU of that hospital, where anybody and everybody ,was allowed to enter at any time; ofcourse thankfully for me, for my selfish reason, that my day could not start without seeing her. And so must, have been the case for all others who kept peeping, entering all the while. Ten days gone, and not a sign of improvement, and rather I could see she was deteriorating, wither breathing being so laborious for her, my poor 'Billy'.

Awaiting the lab results of the most simple tests even, days were being wasted. Finally, a call from the U.S. from our 'doctor saab', and it was all, sun and light. Heading for the airport to fetch her, on return journey to the hospital, I was narrating the events or rather the non events.

Ambulance was arranged, bills were paid, discharge or LAMA (left against medical advice) was obtained, my 'Billy' was shifted delicately to the state of the art Ambulance, inspiring confidence and hope. The song in my heart started.

The flashing lights, the screaming sirens and my vision blurred ,by the drops of tears and the drops of rain drizzle outside, I was driving my small omni, following or was it chasing the smooth and sleek giant of an ambulance. I was left trailing,with only the flashing lights being visible

My world was tumbling. Myself just a shadow of my mother, I had yet not outgrown the habit of following her, whining all the time for her company, even till then.

The team of doctors, discussing amongst themselves, myself, not even understanding, like most patients around, various tests were conducted, and fast. One particular test being a cath test. My Billy went through everything . The bright lights all around in the lobby, could not wipe out the dark moments when it was disclosed that there was a blockage in the arteries and same was requiring surgery.

I hated it. I hated the doctors. I did not accept anything. All I knew was the healthy and hard working lady, who never so much as, even agreed to take a mild pain killer or any mild medicine even. And here she was, just a ‘putty’, her will ,her desires ignored. She was convinced, and so was I, and reluctantly, hardly seeing much choice, I gave in.

She went through it bravely. Not a sign of worry or anxiety. We returned home. Happy days were returning, perhaps or maybe not.

Another trip to Shimla. My 'Billy', my favourite sister, my second mother, and her angel like daughter. The rain, the fog, we were all in it.

However she started having symptoms of anxiety. About small nitty-gritty, she started to go on reminding or inquiring. The increased medicines were doing their job. Problems she never faced were happening.

Not that her arteries were perfect. The blockages returned, and this time it was informed, that her kidney function was affected.

ALTERNATIVE REMEDIES

"THE MISTRUST CREATED"

I started administering various effective homoepathic medicines (as advised) to her just taking over the role of my father who was no more. She would often express, how she missed him, but soon she would shed the depressing thought, and be her own vibrant cheerful self.

Unrelented efforts were being made, so as to avoid any increase of allopathic medicines. But that was not to be. Tablets were increasing in number and in size. No one trusted the homoepathic or ayurvedic or any other alternative therapies, though the hospital was keeping on a display ,books on alternative therapies.

Quite surprisingly, the very Senior Consultant nephrologist, who had got his article published about the ill effects of hemodialysis on the very old and very young, prescribed hemodialysis for my 83 year old mother, who was already becoming quite weak from the ill effects of so many medicines. I tried to reason out, as to why hemodialysis, and for that matter why dialysis at all. Why not I be allowed to intensify the alternative medicine like homoepathic, and why not give me an opportunity to avoid dialysis.

THE ROAD TO THE END

Mother was hospitalized, and I was racing against time, as the doctor seemed in undue haste, to start dialysis. I managed to obtain one week time to try out the alternative treatment. On the fourth day itself, the craetenin stopped increasing, though no doubt it was still high. I came rushing to the hospital to plead with everyone concerned and the Senior doctor to stay their hands on dialysis. But to my utter discouragement the first round had been given, and the road to the end had begun!

At that point of time, I had started to wonder as to what had become of the medical profession. Whether it was still a medical profession or it had been reduced to being a medical industry.

The very same senior consultants who were seen to be advocating against the process of dialysis as inadvisable for the children of tender age or for very elderly people, were seen to be advising in favour of it, and this was inspite of the various protests and objections.

There was a kind of haste which could be deduced while I was running from pillar to post, and even alternative medicines brought and administered were showing some results, they were in a rush to start with the dialysis, and once it started, there was no end, and the end was just brought close.

At this point of time, I happened to come across a few articles written by Professor B.M. Hegde, and being specialist in the field, and much honoured and esteemed for his specialized knowledge, surprisingly putting down current status of the medical field so precisely and without any hesitation, that one could have no option but to conclude that, the medical profession is now more of a giant industry, wherein the patients are mere inanimate objects with no sensitivity left for their feelings and emotions, and are victim of these giant machines.

The trend is towards bringing each and every citizen under the medical scanner, and gradually step by step to introduce a kind of phobia and constant checking of blood sugar level, blood pressure and with the result that on one or the other occasion, he would fall prey to the tables, available in abundance, with one simple deficiency, or excess, leading upto thousands of complications.

Some of the extracts from the said articles sound as so actual, and nothing could be more, near the truth, atleast inasmuch as what I also observed and felt through the agony of my mother.

After seeing the condition of my mother, what I exactly felt was very accurately expressed in the articles authored by Great Prof. B.M. Hegde the extracts of some of which I take liberty to quote here.

THE SICKNESS INDUSTRY

Health care, as it is called and advertised, is, in fact, an industry based on human misery and/or sickness. No industry wants its business to go down in the interest of its stake holders. Naturally, the establishment does not want sickness to disappear!

Therefore, the so called health care has become a health scare industry to get more business.

Fear is the key to most, if not all, illnesses. By creating fear in the minds of the people, the industry is disease mongering.

The new science of biology and medicine makes it easier for patients to have less expensive but more effective healing methods. The conventional disease model is outdated.

We will have to go in for whole person healing. There have been attempts to authenticate cheaper healing methods using hard scientific yard sticks. Our group, The World Academy of Authentic Healing Sciences, is in the forefront in this area. We have a ground of fifteen world class scientists helping us to authenticate the healing methods even in other alternate systems of medicine.

Future is for an integrated system which retains some of the corrective surgical methods from modern medicine along with selected emergency care methods. Preserving the health of the well should be the backbone of the future system. That was the core of Ayurveda–Swasthashya Swaastha Rakshitham–preserve the health of the well using immune boostes, the leading Light here is the sunlight itself. Now that we know that individual cells, which work identically are at the root of our illness and/or wellness we could take advantage of energy, known and/or occult to correct the defects. Our group has succeeded in getting any cell (tissue) damage corrected by using electromagnetic energy of a particular frequency with remarkable success. Other groups elsewhere are also working with many other simple, inexpensive method to heal the sick. Of course, the multi–trillion dollar sickness industry will try and sabotage the efforts for their survival. We have to work hard to show them how they could still do business in the new future healing arena by modifying their thinking and their dubious methods. As these methods have come after the so–called modern medicine, I prefer to call the future healing methods as Meta–medicine, on the lines of meta–physics. Time has come to go back to our ancient methods of healing the sick and not curing his/her pathology. We have come one full circle. The wellness model needs to be popularized among younger generation who are unfortunately sold to the western methods of junk food, chemicals loaded soft drinks and some stimulants in addition. This needs de-schooling the whole society as they are, at the moment, oblivious to their surroundings that are being completely vitiated by vested interests for their benefit.

Food is one's medicine and medicine is one's food is an old but, true adage. Indian food habits have been much healthier, certainly for Indians, but also for others. The agricultural methods need to be indigenized using organic forming. Drinking water and sanitation in our villages and city slums will have to be specially strengthened. The future health care system should be inclusive, taking even the poorest along with us. Today modern medicine hardly reaches less than one per cent of the population. Medical education needs to have major radical surgery to make it need based for our country and relevant to our needs. Medical schools should lay stress on the scientifically authenticated healing methods of other systems as much as of western medicine.

Share our similarities, celebrate our differences.

– M.Scott Peck.

Best Medical Advice: "DON'T"

Prof. B.M. Hegde

"One of the first duties of the physician is to educate the masses not to take medicine," is one of the many brilliant sayings of Sir William Osler.

In the twenty first century, I could only echo that great sentiment as a truism, despite all the tall talk about the "so called" evidence based medicine.

Napoleon Bonaparte went one step further, but one could argue that he was not a physician. Napoleon was at the receiving end of such a medical practice in Persia where he died.

"Medicine is a collection of uncertain prescriptions, the results of which, taken collectively, are more fatal than useful to mankind". Napoleon, though, was more accurate scientifically today. Latest science says that uncertainty is the only certainty in the world. This is truer in medical science, if there is one. A proverb is a short sentence based on long experience. If that were so, this one from Voltaire takes the cake; "The art of medicine consists in amusing the patient while nature cures the disease".

Time and again I had written that our evidence base has been built on loose sand. Of course, no one seems to take it seriously. They would have, if it had any financial interest behind it.

The present Randomised Controlled Trials and linear relations help generate billions of dollars in chemical therapeutics even if that results in thousands dying of our efforts directly or indirectly.

A study by researchers in an US university of the placebo based RCTs did show that the contents of the placebo capsule, which need not legally be made known to the regulating agencies were very potent substances that would show the Company drug as very effective in comparison.

To cite an example, anti–diabetic d rugs are compared with sugar filled placebo capsules! Many such glaring criminal activities have come to light now in the field of "Evidence based medicine" of today.

Recently, I had a message from one of my old students who is a leading dermatologist in India doing innovative research in his area. "I always wondered when I used to listen to you during my student days and respected your views all along. In dermatology evidence is found only in 28% of published studies. All molecular biology companies come with an offer to give authorship if we buy their equipment for our laboratory. Doesn't that mean that moist molecular biology studies are prototype and try to find out how what is known fits into their studies?"

Foundations of our evidence in modern medicine like the statistical risk calculations, (especially the relative risk reductions in place of absolute risk reductions that are sold to gullible doctors in most of the "scientific" articles without mentioning the NNT figures) and, the RCTs, which have no true science base, are very shaky, indeed. We need to have a new science of man, which is sadly missing in this whole bargain.

Physics changed in 1925 and there is no more physics, but we still use the same old physics laws for our statistics. Matter is not made up of matter. Matter and energy are interchangeable. Human molecules communicate with one another which can now be documented through the photon lights emitted from each DNA.

What is the science base of our reductionism, organ based specialization and our reliance on Mendelian inheritance? Instead of trying to rehash the existing evidence base it is better to think of a new evidence base for health and illness. Health is a state where each human body cell is in sync with other cells.

Illness is when this communication breaks down. We need a new non–linear, holistic, dynamic, scientific base for further medical research. Nature has provided a robust repair mechanism inside the human system which has been weakened by our modern life style. Even though both Claude Bernard and Louis Pasteur did note that the "terrain is more important than the seed" when we have gone a whole hog on the seed, risk factors, and what have you. Modern medicine has forgotten the essence of illness care which is basically to strengthen the terrain.

Indian Ayurveda and many other complementary systems stress just that fact to strengthen one's immune system. Ayurveda has many immune boosting modalities in its armamentarium. Many simple methods which have stood the test of time are being forgotten now, thanks to the brainwashing of the masses through mass media advertisements about the wrong approaches to keep one healthy. The leading one among them is goading people to have regular "health" check up. Nothing could be more dangerous than that to apparently healthy people.

When one is healthy one should NEVER ever go for a check up. Common man will have the doubt as to how/s/he could know about health. One is healthy when one has, (a) enthusiasm to work, and, (b) enthusiasm to be compassionate.

One of the ancient exercises could be the most potent modern medicine–a daily walk if one is not a physical labourer.

Universal love is another life giving elixir.

Latest science says that uncertainty is the only certainty in the world. This is truer in medical science, if there is one. A proverb is a short sentence based on long experience.

If that were so, this one from Voltaire takes the cake: "The art of medicine consists in amusing the patient while nature cures the disease".

Time and again I had written in responses to the journal as also in my articles elsewhere that our evidence base has been built on loose sand.

Of course, no one seems to take in seriously. They would have, if it had any financial interest behind it.

The present Randomised Controlled Trials and linear relations help generate billions of dollars in chemical therapeutics even if that results in thousands dying of our efforts directly or indirectly.

We need a new non–linear, holistic, dynamic, scientific base for future medical research. Nature has provided a robust repair mechanism inside the human system which has been weakened by our modern life style. Even though both Claude Bernard and Louis Pasteur did note that the "terrain is more important than the seed" we have gone whole hog on the seed, risk factors, and what have you. Modern medicine has forgotten the essence of illness care which is basically to strengthen the terrain.

Indian Ayurveda and many other complementary systems stress just that fact to strengthen one's immune system.

Ayurveda has many immune boosting modalities in its armamentarium. Many simple methods which have stood the test of time are being forgotten now, thanks to the brain washing of the masses through mass media advertisements about the wrong approaches to keep one healthy. The leading one among them is goading people to have regular "health" check up. Nothing could be more dangerous than that to apparently health people.

When one is healthy one should NEVER ever go for a check. Common man will have the doubt as to how s/he could know about health. One is healthy when one has:

- enthusiasm to work and
- enthusiasm to be compassionate

One of the ancient exercises could be the most potent modern medicine – a daily walk if one is not a physical labourer. Universal love is another life giving elixir.

They are After your Wealth Not Health, Mind You!

Prof. B.M. Hegde

"Give all thou canst; high Heaven rejects the lore of nicely-calculated less or more."

- William Wordsworth. (1770-1850)

I was at a function a few days ago when an agitated young medico came in a great hurry to see me. He had called my house first and then came to the venue directly. I asked him gently as to who he was and what the provocation for his acute anxiety state.

He slowly opened up. He was a student for a government medical college and had secured a merit seat for doing MD in general medicine. As he had a few months time to join his course, he took a temporary job in a teaching hospital in Mangalore.

That morning a middle–aged man had come to the casualty with chest pain since morning. This doctor reached the conclusion that the pain was not due to myocardial ischaemia (angina pain) and was in the process of allaying the patient's anxiety. The latter was about to go when one of the senior cardiac surgeons walked in. the cardiac surgeon saw this young doctor about to send the patient away.

He took the young medico to the adjoining room and told him that this was not the method of disposing of anyone with any kind of chest pain. He said: "first find out the patient's personal details like, his financial status, whether he has medical insurance or a Govt. or corporate job that reimburse his medical bills etc. In case the patient comes from a poor strata of society what the young medico was about to do was right but NOT for a rich man or for one who has a god father to pay for him.

The young doctor was advised to reinvestigate the patient using all the available tests in the hospital (if the patient can afford) and then asked for a coronary angiogram as he might have some blocks in the coronary arteries needing a bypass graft. The young man was told that that is how corporate hospitals work these days.

The cultural shock was too much for the young man to bear. He was so confused that he wanted to quit the medical profession if it is this inhuman. To take a final decision on what to do, he went to see one of his teachers. Looking at this young man's state of mind, his teacher who happened to be an old friend of mine, directed him to see me and gave my address, etc. That is how he came to me.

He was caught in an ethical dilemma. Little did he realize that the medical fraternity today, especially in the fee–for–service system has become a corporate monstrosity. He was innocent and believed in medical ethics and was keen to do service to the less fortunate after becoming a doctor. All those dreams and the castles in the air he was building about his future seemed to come down and collapse suddenly.

It took me nearly half an hour to get the medico to reality and convince him that it is not good to run away from a problem but to stand and fight it. It is the minority like him that can change the set up. People like him are the hope of the suffering humanity. He agreed with me and was quite composed when he left. He promised me that he will study for his MD with greater vigour with a resolve to stand up to be counted in the fight against falling moral standards in the profession. May his tribe increase!.

I asked the young man as to how he was so sure that his patient did not need bypass surgery. He was up–to–date, even though he was only a fresh MBBS. He told me that the only study large enough to give an opinion on bypass surgery, not funded by vested interests, the CASS study, showed that 84% patients did not get even a day's extension of life expectancy while the remaining 16% got some relief.

There are only TWO scientific indications for bypass surgery – intractable chest pain despite the best medical management and severally compromised left ventricular function. Neither of them was present in this man.

In all other cases bypass surgery could increase the risk of a future heart attack, quadruple the risk of acute stroke, have 47% long term resultant cognitive defects, some of them quite incapacitating.

Bypass does not even reduce the risk of sudden death due to malignant arrhythmias. He concluded by saying that he has saved one human life by sending the man away. I was speechless.

The moral of this true story is what Professor Harlan Krumholz of Yale University wrote in the New England Journal of Medicine (NEJM 1997; 336:1523) about cardiac interventions: "cardiac procedures bring in billions of dollars in cash for doctors, hospitals and the instrument manufacturers, in addition to television interviews. The procedures are done mainly to get those benefits and not to help patients in the USA."

This is the long and short of the present–day medical economics. It is not about doing good, damn it! In 1823, James Wakely, a young MD and member of the House of Commons, thought that the London doctors at that time were a bunch of "incompetent, corrupt, and nepotistic" humans that looked like an abscess on the body of the profession.

The medical profession, in the words of Hillary Butler, a medical journalist, has become "a corporate monstrosity"! very sad!.

The Healers and the Killers

G.A. Mathew

According to WHO statistics, more than a crore and twenty lakh people die every year due to heart disease. This number is much higher than all those people who perished in all the wars fought in the history of the world. In the developed countries, it remains the number one killer. This happens despite the most expensive medications and the most sophisticated surgeries.

Cardiology seems to be obsessed with high cholesterol, the biggest risk factor according to modern medicine. To combat this, it has an array of cholesterol lowering drugs, the stains. They have become the most–widely prescribed class of drugs in history. These stain drugs bring in more revenue to pharmaceutical companies than any other class of medicine known.

Ten such pharma companies at the top of Fortune 500 companies have a higher total income than all the other 490 companies put together, says Marcia Angell of the New England Journal of Medicine, in her book, The Truth About The Drug Companies. Despite their mountains of tablets intended to lower high cholesterol, the heart disease is assuming epidemic proportions. Obviously, cardiology is after the wrong enemy, the wrong cause.

Surgical procedures such as angioplasty and bypasses are no effective solutions.

According to Dr. Norton Hadler, M.D., angioplasty has no justification whatsoever, 95% of all bypasses too are useless because, in a vast majority of them, the disease appears again. It is like the repeated clogging of the drainage channel even after thorough cleaning.

Angioplasty is meaningless and dangerous. It is a procedure in which a balloon on the tip of a catheter is used to open blockages. Dr. Julian Whitaker, M.D., states that, "there is never any reason for anyone to have angioplasty; it is a dangerous procedure which has no scientific validation."

Studies comparing angioplasty with other non–surgical procedures show that patients treated with angioplasty, virtually always fare worse. "There is a higher death rate, higher heart attack rate, and in general, a repeat surgery rate. This procedure will always be an unproven, expensive and dangerous gimmick that became an accepted therapy based on self–serving `presumption' only," adds Dr.Whitaker.

Dr.Whitaker castigates the dishonest cardiac surgeons who strike terror into the heart of the patient and his/her dear ones insisting that immediate surgery only can save the patient. He assures in a prestigious medical journal that 98.4% of heart patients, advised for immediate surgery, will be fine without any such surgery.

Dr. Thomas Graboys of Harvard Medical School, conducted a review study. This study shed light on a heart hoax, a secret agenda, perpetrated in the hallowed heart hospitals. He methodically reevaluated 168 patients recommended for angioplasty, after angiogram. He was shocked to find that only six of the 168 patients were proper candidates for that costly, risky procedure. Dr. Michael Ozner, M.D., calls such unethical commercialization the great American heart hoax.

You will be startled to hear that the routine surgical treatment of heart disease is harming moré people than it is helping. This daring statement is made on the basis of arguments by an eminent doctor himself. His disturbing finding is based on a series of scientific studies starting from 1977 that all show the same thing: compared to non–surgical therapies, surgery almost always does more damage than good.

Dr. Whitaker points to a comparative study of conservative vs. invasive treatment on patients who had had mild heart attacks.

Los Angeles Times (March 20, 1997) brought it to the attention of the public in a front page article. The results of the study were again clear and unequivocal: the immediate use of an invasive strategy, which mostly lead to angioplasty and bypass surgery not only did not help patients but increased the in–hospital death rate by 71%.

The guiding lights to doctors in the USA are the American College of Cardiology and the American Heart Association. For over a decade and half, these outfits have recommended that patients with mild heart attack undergo immediate catheterisation, or angiography. This is a procedure that involves threading a catheter into the arteries of the heart in order to see the location and severity of blockages in those arteries.

This leads to a dramatic increase in the use of bypass surgery and angioplasty, because physicians then try to open up observed blockages to prevent heart attacks or death. As some one said, if the only tool a man has is a hammer he sees every problem as the head of a nail and hits.

Surgeons find every reason to conduct a surgery. There are no scientific studies to indicate that "invasive strategy" is best for patients, but that has not prevented the heart industry from going ahead on the presumption that it is.

William E. Boden, MD, organized a study to test the validity of the recommendations of immediate invasive action on patients with mild heart attacks. He followed 920 patients, who had had mild heart attacks, for two and a half years. 458 of these received medications. They used simple non–invasive tests (like treadmill) in monitoring their condition. The remaining 462 underwent catheterization (angiography) followed by bypass surgery or angioplasty in 45% of the patients.

The results were astounding. In the first nine days, 21 of the patients in the "invasive strategy group" died, compared to only six in the other group. At the end of two and a half years, 80 patients in the invasive group had died, compared to only 59 of those in the conservative group, as overall increase in death rate of 36%.

At no stage was there any evidence that an invasive strategy did anything but increase the death rate. The truth is proclaimed loud and clear: today's increasing invasive diagnostic techniques and surgical procedures for heart disease are a hoax.

The physicians bent on doing them may try to justify them. But the risk and futility are as clear as day light. An elephant is there in front of them, but they cannot see it at all because of a strange form of cataract!

Dr. Dwight Lundell, the eminent heart surgeon, did not hesitate to throw away the surgical knife, when he became convinced that surgery would not be the answer.

He recommends life style change and nutritional supplements to solve the heart disease problem. His book, The Cure for Heart Disease, and his e–book, The Great Cholesterol Lie, expose the meaninglessness of surgery and statin drugs. As a heart surgeon, his daily fee was Rs.50 lakh, but now he is happy with recommending supplements worth only Rs.50. Yes, the steam of love is still relentlessly flowing in the wasteland!

"Surgery is always second best. If you can do something else, it's better", said the renowned heart surgeon Dr. John Kirklin of Mayo Clinic. Let us hear what Dr.Michael Ozner, M.D., (board–certified cardiologist and Fellow of both the American Heart Association and the American College of Cardiology) says in his book, The Great American Heart Hoax: "Three major studies performed in the late 1970s and early 1980s clearly proved that for the majority of patients, bypass surgery is no more effective than conservative medical treatment. A majority of patients who underwent bypass surgery did not live significantly longer or have fewer heart attacks than those who did not undergo surgery".

He adds that, "The studies on angioplasty delivered even worse news: angioplasty didn't show any benefit either". It may have justification if the main blocked artery is opened in the midst of a heart attack. Quoting a study, he says that "angioplasty did not reduce the risk of heart attack or death among study subjects – it actually increased it!"

Stents (devices inserted into the artery with plaque to allow increased blood flow) popularised by the heart industry, are not only useless but harmful, according to Dr.Ozner. he quotes a study and says that, "stent placement in the occluded artery responsible for the recent heart attack did not reduce the occurrence of repeat heart attack or heart failure.

In fact, there was an increase in repeat heart attacks among patients receiving stents during the study's four years of follow–up. What seemed to make sense – opening a blocked artery with a stent following a heart attack – was conclusively found not to be beneficial, and in some respects even detrimental".

Honest cardiologists think that surgical procedures in patients not in the midst of heart attack have no justification. The problem with angioplasty and stents is a gradual return of blockage to the cleared arteries. "Roughly one–third of the patients who received stents had a return of their coronary blockage within six months."

Hear Dr. Ozner: "Millions of these new stents were inserted – again, without sufficient clinical study. And soon it became apparent that coated stents could result in a catastrophic complication: sudden, unpredictable clotting that occurred at the stent site and led to heart attack or sudden cardiac death, especially in patients who either stopped or were taken off their blood thinners."

But they are mighty glad to point out the little speck of dust in others' eyes. The physicians point an accusing, venomous finger, and state that "there is no scientific evidence" for vitamin therapy or naturotherapy or any of the alternative therapies.

But there are scientific evidences galore that can perfectly satisfy world–class scientists and Nobel Laureates. But these prejudiced ones pretend not to see them or refuse to see them.

These physicians control the American Heart Association and the American College of Cardiology. For the past one and a half decades, they have recommended immediate catheterisation for the treatment of patients with mild heart attacks without any scientific grounding whatsoever. They will keep harping on the same strings to please their masters.

How is it possible that doctors still regularly recommend stents and surgery, promising it will "fix" their patients in the face of so much evidence to the contrary? Will all the waters of the seven seas wash their conscience clean?

The plaque appears as a strange foreign substance to the immune system of the body. It tries to get rid of it. If it succeeds in the effort, the plaque will burst and spill the content into the blood stream. As soon as it happens, the blood clots. The blood clot can result in partial or complete blockage of the artery. Complete blockage leads to heart attack.

Not every plaque ruptures. Some are perfectly stable with a thick fibrous, calcified cap. So the bigger the plaque, the less likely is it to burst. A big plaque becoming bigger and bigger, and eventually restricting blood flow to cause chest pain is a possibility, but not always a fact.

The real threat can be from small, unstable plaques which have no thick, fibrous, calcified caps. We are blissfully unaware of many a rupture in our coronary arteries. Our wonderful body dissolves the resulting clots. Only when it fails, it results in heart attack or stroke. The comforting news is that proper life styles and nutritional supplements can boost the body's defenses.

We have seen that the large plaques seldom rupture and result in blood clot. This important point is often overlooked. Dishonest doctors often point to the large, scary plaques, and insist on stent or bypass to the confused, bewildered patients and their relatives in their hour of agony.

Another very important point they try to hide from the patients is that large blockages often foster the development of collateral blood vessels – new vessels that spontaneously develop, forging a path around the blockage.

Like water in a stream that has been partially dammed, blood naturally tries to find a way around any blockage in a blood vessel. Blood travels through tiny blood vessels that spring to life, circumvent the plaque, and then reconnect with the original path, until the path is fully developed.

As a result, the heart muscle is able to receive the oxygenated blood it needs, despite the blockage in the original vessel. Michael Ozner, M.D., calls this a natural heart bypass. How many patients hear about this incredible ability of our own bodies from the doctors?

Cardiologists and heart surgeons scare the hell out of the patients and `frighten' them into heart surgery. It leaves psychological scars that last forever. If you say `NO' to recommendations of angiogram or surgery, expect a plethora of fear–inspiring scenarios. Surgeons are known to use phrases like "you are a walking time bomb," "you could go at any minute," "you might not make it to next Christmas," "the next heart beat may be your last," and "you are living on borrowed time."

Harvard cardiologist and Nobel Laureate Bernard Lown, M.D., calls these "words that maim." In his extraordinary book, The Lost Art of Healing, he lists many examples of phrases like the above, used by uncaring or manipulative physicians. Doctors are doctors anywhere; some are good and caring, but a good many are after your money and not your health.

Dr. Whitaker says that this frightening technique generates hundreds of thousands of unnecessary procedures or operations. He wonders why a class action suit has not been brought against the entire heart industry, including the American Heart Association and the American College of Cardiology.

Dr. Whitaker calculates that these meaningless, senseless procedures cause 33,000 deaths per year in the USA. These unfortunate patients do not die in the throes of heroic measures by doctors to save their lives. They die from surgical procedures.

It is truly tragic that many of them are quite healthy, and did not even need the procedure (operation) to begin with. The 33,000 deaths in the US alone are roughly equal to the annual number of deaths attributed to AIDS. Can we take that the Indian doctors are more caring and honest than the American doctors? God save us because they will not!

There is good news! A new cardiology without costly medicines and surgeries has been revealed by Dr. Linus Pauling, the only person in history to be awarded two unshared Nobel prizes.

According to him, the present heartless, mystified cardiology promoted by the greedy pharma lobby, can be likened to Much Ado About Nothing of the immortal Shakespearean play. All the fear, fuss and noise about heart disease, all the helpless submission to costly surgical procedures, all the pitiful guttering of the personality of the patients, and all the prohibitively high expenses are due to our ignorance of the real cause of the problem. A giant lobby works incessantly to keep us ignorant. The real cause of heart disease is deceptively simple. So unbelievably simple is the answer also.

If the natural therapy for heart disease that Dr.Linus Pauling taught becomes widely known, the whole heart industry of today will instantly come crashing like the once–imposing twin towers of the

World Trade Center; and the cardiologists will go begging for their daily bread!

The revolutionary discovery of Dr.Linus Pauling and others which sometime ago shook the world, is that heart disease is caused by scurvy. This is the disease from which sailors of old died in their long sea voyages. When they lacked vitamin C in their diet –from fresh vegetables and fruits – their blood vessels degenerated, decayed; they died miserably with internal bleeding.

Dr. Pauling staked his reputation on this life–changing theory. He proclaimed to the whole world: "Now I have gotten to the point where I think we can get almost complete control of cardiovascular disease, heart attacks and strokes."

Heart disease remains the dreaded number one killer only because the pharma–dominated doctors refuse to recognize this momentous theory. They stand to lose a lot. So they fight it tooth and nail. Most of them are ignorant of such an important scientific breakthrough.

In their complete submission to the medical–surgical mode of interventions they fail to see anything worthwhile outside their realm. They surely are the very cream of society. But they dread the possibility that they may after all be wrong. What if all that they learned and believed in, came crashing down like nine pins! Naturally, they are afraid to seek the truth, and face the truth if they find it. Some children are afraid of the dark. But how on earth these educated, elite, highly accomplished individuals mortally fear the light!

"(This is a chapter from the upcoming book: POWERFUL NATURAL REMEDIES for Heard Disease, Cancer, AIDS and Other Diseases)

World without Medicines

Prof. B.M. Hegde

"The groundwork of all happiness is health."

-James Leigh Hunt (1784-1859)

The latest issue of Reader's Digest has an article with the above title where the author seems to be frightened of a future world without medicines as the drug companies will no longer be interested to make good drugs if rules allow medicines to be manufactured and sold with generic names. Generic drugs remove the present day power of the Pharma lobby to sell the same medicines with their patent for anywhere between 1000–5000 timed the cost!

I pity the author, Katherine Eban, who obviously is a non–medical person and looks like an agent of the pharmaceutical corporate monstrosity. I, as a doctor and medical teacher of more than half a century's experience, am daily praying for a world without reductionist chemical medicines for the good of mankind.

The leading cause of death today seems to be the infamous adverse drug reactions of those reductionist molecules.

Most, if not all, diseases begin in the human mind as that is the only reality in this world of biocentrism. This world is created by our consciousness.

In this context there is no room for any reductionist thinking. "Positive sciences do not answer the question "why", wrote Nobel Laureate physiologist Charles Sherrington. They can only answer "how"?

Let us take a common example of a ghost of that Cholesterol as a disease. If your cholesterol goes up no one asks or answers the question why does our body cholesterol go up while it is being manufactured in our liver for our own survival? We have a limited reductionist thinking–cholesterol is up, it needs to be brought down!

We create drugs–one of the best money spinners–which create misery by their side effects.

Cholesterol has many functions in the body. Trillions of cells in our body have their cell membrane made up of cholesterol.

Billions of cells age and die every day and billions of new ones are replaced needing lots of cholesterol for good health. cholesterol is needed to manufacture steroids, or cortisone–like hormones, including vitamin D and the sex hormones testosterone, estrogen and cortisone.

This in turn controls a myriad of bodily functions. Bile acids are manufactured in the liver with the help of cholesterol. Bile acids are essential for digestion and absorption of fat–soluble vitamins such as vitamin A, D, E and K. Cholesterol is needed for the formation of the myelin sheath, a neuron consisting of fat–containing cells that insulate the axon from electrical activity. This ensures proper functioning of our brain by aiding route of electrical impulses.

The absence of cholesterol might lead to loss of memory and difficulty in focusing. Cells cannot talk to each other without the help of cholesterol. Such a vital substance, 80% of it being produced in our own liver, cannot be lowered forcefully by drugs without serious collateral damage.

Looking holistically the body produces excess cholesterol only when it needs it badly! When one needs more steroids, bile acids, myelin, and cortisol, liver pours in more cholesterol into the circulation.

Steroids and cortisol go up when one is in the fright–flight–fight mode! Anger, jealousy, fear, greed, hostility, pride and super ego produce the fight–fright–flight state. The latter is needed in a dangerous situation like when you see a tiger in a forest to run away, but not on a chronic basis. If one is in that dangerous mode on a daily basis the cholesterol goes up seriously.

Similarly, overeating, especially fatty food and fatty neat demands more bile acids for digestion and the liver responds by producing extra cholesterol to assist in the making of fatty acids in the liver. Sedentary living does not encourage cholesterol catabolism either.

When the question "why" does the cholesterol go up in the first place is viewed with (w) holistic glasses, the foolish (reductionist) need for drugs to lower clean hands disappears. All that one needs to do is to get into the parasympathetic mode in daily life with Yoga, pranayaama, daily exercise and moderation in eating which together would eventually obviate the need for high cholesterol production in the liver. One can see the double whammy here.

The extra work for the liver to manufacture extra cholesterol for the body's needs in the fight–flight–fright mode is removed saving the liver from chromic damage while the need for the deadly anti–cholesterol drugs disappear totally.

One can, at the same time, enjoy a proper meal like any one else as long as one remains within limits. No need to shun any food including fats in moderation.

The immune system, the body's inner healer, works wonders in every situation where the body physiology goes astray as long as we live sensibly in tune with nature. The world without (reductionist) medicines will be a boon to mankind. Herbal medicines are good in the unlikely event that the immune system needs assistance.

The greedy drug lobby could explore that area for making their living in peace while providing good herbal medicines produced with good manufacturing practice!

"A vigorous five–mile walk will do more good for an unhappy but otherwise healthy adult than all the medicine and psychology in the world."

Paul Dudley White (1886-1973) – an American physician and cardiologst

Medical Scare System

Prof. B.M. Hegde

"Of all the fears of the world, sometimes the worst are your own fears."

-Rudyard Kippling

Our greatest achievement in modern medicine has been the success in making the world populace mortally afraid of diseases and death. Hypochondriasis has gone up exponentially since modern hi-tech medicine learnt the "art" of advertising both the morbid side of illnesses and our capacity to "drag people even from the jaws of death." In short, we have taken medicine, a healthy coming together of two human beings the sick and his saviour in mutual trust, into a big business and gone to the market place.

Our deifying ourselves has exposed us to the vagaries of consumer society of fault finding and law suits for negligence. Just read this letter from a friend of mine to find out how fear mongering goes on daily.

"I' m a regular reader of Money life and a big fan of your columns on health. Thank you for sharing your wealth of knowledge with us readers. I know you're not a big fan of western drugs, and can foresee more and more "diseases" being treated with simple herbal holistic drugs of the east.

However, I'm asking this question due to widespread confusion on this issue. I'm about to get married in March and based on my limited online knowledge, recommended my fiancée to take the HIV vaccine shots. Online blogs tell me that this vaccine prevents many forms of cancer in females like cervical, anal, vaginal and vulvar. It also prevents certain STDs for both males and females. Also, I am told that this vaccine is supposed to be taken by girls before they turn 25.

Accordingly, she consulted two doctors. Both advised her to go ahead with the vaccination. But she later came to know of a case in her city wherein a girl got herself vaccinated but the vaccine had massive side-effects. There is a general lack of awareness about this vaccine in India and many doctors also don't guide us properly. Could you please shed some light on the vaccine? It would be of great help to us and others. Thanks for your time."

You see the scare mongering. We have learnt this from big businesses, the biggest being the drug industry. Vaccine business is a gold mine as the clientele is the whole world while drugs treating diseases have limited market. We now advertise our medicines and even ourselves in the media. We, of course, take the Hippocratic oath only to become hypocrites soon after.

Doctors are educated by the drug companies; they do it intentionally. Now the cat is out of the bag.

The British Parliamentary Committee on drug companies has this report just released:

“Drug companies have “routinely and legally” withheld the results of medical trials from doctors, researchers and patients for decades, MPs have said. In a damning report, the Public Accounts Committee said it was of “extreme Concern” that about half of all trial results for medicines available on the global market were not subject to public and independent scrutiny. Warning that doctors and patients are being “undermined” in their ability to make informed decisions on treatment, the committee called on the Government to act to ensure that the results of all clinical trials of every medicine currently being prescribed are made available.

The report will significantly increase pressure on the world’s pharmaceutical giants to commit to full transparency over clinical trials.

Critics have accused “big Pharma” of systematically putting profits before patients, withholding data that might undermine confidence in their blockbuster drugs.

MPs said that "trials which gave a favourable verdict" were "about twice as likely to be published as trials giving unfavourable results."

Dr. Ben Goldacre who gave evidence to the committee, told that the public had been given "false reassurance" by the pharmaceutical industry and the medical establishment for at least 20 years.

"Patients suffer and die unnecessarily because of this," he said. "It's very common that we are persuaded to use the less effective of the available treatments because of withheld trial results.

The Public Accounts Committee said it was "disturbed" by claims that regulators did not have access to all the available trial data on the anti-viral drug Tamiflu. There was "limited evidence and widespread disagreement among regulators and other bodies internationally on whether [it] confers any benefits on complications and mortality". Department of Health reviewed whether to spend a further £49m on stockpiling Tamiflu.

Common man goes by advertisements of the pharma companies in addition to the pharma lobbyselling those ideas to doctors. Advertisements make one buy things that s/he does not need. The best example is the vaccine referred to in Para above. Dr. Diane Harper who helped develop Gardsil, the HPV vaccine, admitted back in 2009 that the jabs are essentially useless and more dangerous than the very conditions they are hailed as preventing and treating?

That was before the vaccine industry apparently convinced her to change her story. You can read more about the saga here. Dr. Diane Harper, a key developer of Gardasil, is on the record as having cleared her conscience about this fraudulent vaccine, which has been shown to be both ineffective and dangerous, "writes Ethan A Huff of Natural news.

Anyone who goes for a check-up or goes with some vague chest discomfort to a hospital having a cardiac care centre, and if affluent, comes back home with either an angioplasty or bypass surgery. Occasionally, the victim might end up in heaven also.

We make them get panicky by showing them some blocks in the four epicardial vessels that are visualized in the angiogram. The usual conversation goes thus: "Are those dangerous, doctor?" asks the hapless victim. "You are sitting on a volcano which might burst and kill you any time sooner than later," tells the cardiologist.

They do not let the victim go home lest s/he should change the mind. They are told that death might even occur on their way home. What we

DON'T tell them is that these intraluminal blocks rarely kill.

The vulnerable lesions that kill are usually not seen in the angiogram as they are inside the blood vessel wall (intramural) and therefore do not show up as blocks inside the vessel lumen.

Dr. Nortin M. Hadler, Professor of Medicine at the university of North Carolina at Chapel Hill and author of the Last Well Person, feels that bypass surgery in particular, he says, "should have been relegated to the archives 15 years ago. Except in a minority of patients with severe disease, bypass operations don't prolong life or prevent future heart attacks, nor does angioplasty. People often believe that having these procedures fixes the problem, as if a plumber came in and fixed the plumbing with a new piece of pipe," explains Dr. L. David Hillis, Professor of Cardiology at the University of Texas, South-Western Medical School. "But it fundamentally doesn't fix the problem."

The heart surgery programme in the US alone is as $ 100 million business. They thrive on panic mongering. There is compelling evidence that more health care and more aggressive treatment across the complete spectrum of illnesses is not necessarily better.

How do some people get benefit from these interventions? Recently, Harvard Medical School Associate Professor of Medicine, Dr. Roger J. Laham reported on follow-up results of a randomized trial looking at laser surgery to improve blood flow. "Patients who got the surgery had significantly less pain and improved heart function. But so did patients who had a sham operation - the equivalent of a placebo.

After 30 minutes the placebo effect was still there. Scans and other tests showed physiological gains in blood flow among only those who thought they had been operated on."

A similar large placebo effect might explain "most of the benefits that we've seen so far with balloon angioplasty and bypass surgery," Laham Says.

Medical scare system increases illness in society to the benefit of the medical industry; good for the latter in an affluent society.

"Nothing in life is to be feared. It is only to be understood. Now is the time to understand more, so that we may fear less".

- Marie Curie

Cancer, Cancer Everywhere but .....

Prof. B.M. Hegde

"Honesty is the first chapter in the book of wisdom"

- Thomas Jefferson

Fresh air of sanity seems to be blowing in the area of cancer and its management. The word cancer brings goose pimples to many and for the hapless patient who gets labeled thus, it is almost a death warrant.

I had been trying to demystify this area for a very long time without much success. Now I feel even the cancer establishment in the US must have had their conscience prick them.

Recently, in July 2013 eight cancer researchers from the National Cancer Institute met to review the area and came up with quite startling conclusions. They felt that the multitude of so called early cancers, in fact, do not behave like cancers at all and might not even grow for years to come. As such they should not be labelled cancer. They could, instead be called indolent epithelial lesions. Small lumps in the thyroid, breast, lung, and prostate come under this category.

As soon as the report from National Cancer Institute came out there was a small group of "specialists" who came out with their opposition for the new idea. This is a usual phenomenon by the industry.

Way back when the JNC V report on blood pressure management came out, the recommendation was that diuretics are the first line of treatment.

After a month a group of so–called hypertension experts in the USA issued a statement that the recommendations are not in order and Ace inhibitors should have been included in the first line.

In retrospect, the suggestion of experts had been proven wrong. The drug industry is very powerful; it does not want its expensive drugs to be relegated to the background.

They will invent some method of bringing back their drugs to the market. Similar efforts are afoot to get the banned anti diabetic drugs back.

This time round, it might not be that easy to reverse the new cancer statement from the National Cancer Institute as it has the backing of the whole institute, including its Nobel Laureate Director, Dr.Varmus. The new wisdom from the NCI will go a long way in helping poor patients who otherwise would all be having the inhuman three pronged attack on their innocent lesions with the wrong label of cancer.

This brings me back to my favourite topic of cancer screening. There is nothing called early cancer as all cancers start as mutated rogue body cells and take years to manifest as symptomatic cancer. The vast majority of them die out as such and never reach the stage of real cancer.

So if we detect these cells in their growing phase, we might give treatment unnecessarily. The lay public, the philanthropic NGOs, and the doctors need to be educated in this area not to waste their time and money screening for cancers in asymptomatic stage. Experience with prostate cancer and PSA testing (which the US government has now banned) has given us enough data not to interfere in cancers in the asymptomatic stage.

We have lived here for hundreds of thousands of years not with the help of doctors and screening. If we were to believe that the modern medical establishment is the one that is keeping us healthy and well, we are mistaken.

It is the body's wisdom that keeps us going. Any disease in its asymptomatic stage is being managed by our inbuilt doctor, the immune system. It is only in the unlikely event of the immune system failing, do doctors come into the picture to "cure rarely, comfort mostly, but to console always."

This brings us to the arena of pre-cancer, pre-diabetes, pre –hypertension, etc. all these are only myths and detecting them early to treat them at that stage might be counter–productive. The risk factor theory, much touted as a great idea, has been shown to be a wrong lead. The famous MRFIT (multiple risk factor interventional trial), which spent millions of tax payer's dollars at the end of 25 years observation showed that there are no risk factors at all. The study turned out to be a boondoggle.

It also showed that while the so called risk factors (surrogate end points) could be controlled by interventions, the final risk of premature death remains intact (real end point). If the drug companies want to make lots of money, I have a suggestion to them. Death is a risk for everyone who gets born! Why not create a new risk factor called pre-death syndrome and treat everyone born with drugs to keep them alive permanently?

There are more than 3500 species of mammals that live by nature depending on their immune systems for survival while it is only one mammal, man, who recently has come to believe that it is outside interventions that keep us alive. With this conviction human kind is the only one that starts to poison their offsprings with nearly 30 mercury laced vaccines as soon as they are born, give them drugs from childhood to control all and sundry ailments, look for outside intervention every time something goes amiss, and even when they become old and disabled they are wheeled into the Intensive Care Units to be tortured till they die!

ICUs have become a necessary evil for the rich and the powerful as an exit route while it is the ICUs that form ninety per cent of hospital profits in US hospitals by keeping dying patient there during the last ten days of their lives.

When hospitals started in Europe centuries ago, almost all patients who went there went to heaven. This was called hospitalism. Are we going back to that hell again?

Cancer industry is the most profitable and lucrative industry in the sickness care business. Hope Dr. Varmus's efforts to demystify cancer help the common man. People like me do not count at all. I must write to thank him for vindicating my long held belief.

Winston Churchill had said that "in every opinion there are three things that matter–who gives the opinion, how does he give the opinion, and finally what is the opinion? Of the three, Churchill felt, that the last is the least important. Now that a Nobel Laureate medical scientist gives the opinion that a village doctor like me has been giving for decades, the latter gets vindicated in India as we believe in the titles from the west, that too a Nobel, which makes most of us drool.

"No legacy is so rich as honesty."

- William Shakespeare

My articles on cancer over the years have been stressing one important truth that many of the so called early cancers are not cancer at all. My friends and, even some of my old students, have been upset and were cursing me. This Monday (July 27th 2013) was a great day for me when a group of scientists from the National Cancer Institute published their finding after a meeting where they seem to have discovered that truth that had dawned on me decades ago making me an object of ridicule in the eyes of my colleagues.

Their recommendations were published in the Journal of the American Medical Association. Some premalignant conditions, like the one that affects the breast called ductal carcinoma in situ, they feel, should be renamed to exclude the word "carcinoma" so that patients are less frightened and less likely to seek what may be unneeded and potentially harmful treatments that can include the surgical removal of the breast. "They also suggested that many of the lesions detected during breast, prostate, thyroid, lung and other cancer screenings should not be called cancer at all but should be reclassified as "indolent lesions of epithelial origin."

"we need a 21st –century definition of cancer instead of a 19th–century definition of cancer, which is what we've been using," said Dr. Otis W. Brawley, the chief medical officer for the American Cancer Society.

The impetus for this call for change must have come from the growing concern of some doctors, scientists and patient advocates that millions of men and women are "undergoing needless and sometimes disfiguring and harmful treatments for premalignant and cancerous lesions that are so slow growing they are unlikely to ever cause harm."

The recent routine screening using modern gadgets has increased the cancer diagnosis so much that overdiagnosis and overtreatment causing misery for millions is so common to merit urgent action.

"we're still having trouble convincing people that the things that get found as a consequence of mammography and P.S.A. testing and other screening devices are not always malignancies in the classical sense that will kill you," said Dr. Harold Varmus, the Nobel Prize–winning director of the National Cancer Institute. "Just as the general public is catching up to this idea, there are scientists who are catching up, too."

"Ductal carcinoma in situ is not cancer, so why are we calling it cancer?" said Dr. Esserman, who is a professor of surgery and radiology at the University of California, San Francisco.

The demand for changing the name of cancer has precedents. The World Health Organisation in 1998 changed the name of an early–stage urinary tract tumour, removing the word "carcinoma" and calling it "papillary urothelial neoplasia of low malignant potential".

"Changing the language we use to diagnose various lesions is essential to give patients confidence that they don't have to aggressively treat every finding in a scan," Dr. Erasmus said. She went on "the problem for the public is you hear the word cancer, and you think you will die unless you get treated. We should reserve this term `cancer' for those things that are highly likely to cause a problem.:

Today doctors are finding and treating scores of seemingly precancerous lesions and early–stage cancers – like ductal carcinoma in situ, a condition called Barrett's oesophagus, small thyroid tumours and early prostate cancer.

But even after aggressively treating those conditions for years, there has not been a commensurate reduction in invasive cancer, suggesting that overdiagnosis and overtreatment are occurring on a large scale.

The new director of the National Cancer Institute, Nobel Laureate himself, Dr. Varmus, has been proactive in setting the cancer industry's house in order by asking some provocative questions of his colleagues to find ways and means to say which of the present day cancers are slow growing or aggressive using some molecular tests.

"This is a long way from the thinking 20 years ago when you found a cancer cell and felt you had a tremendous risk of dying", Dr. Varmus said.

We have come a long way from the nineteenth century diagnosis of cancer. We need a new twenty–first century diagnosis where only aggressively growing cancers need symptomatic treatment. This boils down to what I have been saying about any disease in general.

"Patient doing well–do not interfere" was William Osler's famous advice in 1905 AD.

I think he is right even today. Pre–cancer, pre–diabetes, pre–hypertension and such fancy ideas have resulted in millions undergoing treatment when it was not needed and might be even dangerous.

In the pre–symptomatic stage no disease could benefit from outside intervention as the immune system is trying its best to correct the problem.

It is only in the unlikely event of the immune system getting over powered do symptoms arise.

That is when we, doctors, do come into the picture to "cure rarely, comfort mostly but to console always."

I am happy that the National Cancer Institute of USA, under the able guidance of its new director, Dr. Varmus, is following a very sensible line of science. My stand has now been vindicated.

In India we need American certificate before any new idea is even looked at. Long live the new science of man for the good of humanity.

"Education leads to enlightenment. Enlightenment opens the way to empathy. Empathy foreshadows reform."- Derrick A. Bell, Faces At The Bottom Of The Well.

Medicine - Too much, Too bad

Prof. B.M. Hegde

"Medical science is making such remarkable progress that soon none of us will be well."

- Aldous Huxley

At long last the West has woken up to the reality that in our reductionist science of medicine, use of chemical drugs of all hues and colours as therapeutic tools has resulted in more sorrow and death than cure or healing! Recently there was a big conference in Hanover organized by the British Medical Journal, Consumer's Reports, and Dartmouth and Bond Universities to look into this problem of too much medicine! The unanimous opinion of the conference participants, of which there were more than six hundred scientists, specialists and pharmaceutical representatives, was that too much medicine is too bad.

Be that as it may, let us look at the down side of too much interventions, too much investigations and too many drugs for even imaginary diseases called pre–disease states.

The area needing urgent attention to reduce this menace, in my opinion, is to leave the well segment of the population alone lest they should become patients for life long drugging without, in the first place, having any illness at all, all because of this screening industry.

Many of my regular readers would know about my relentless campaign to educate the public about the drug menace brought on by the greedy drug industry aided and abetted by the vested interests that stand to benefit from this human misery.

Routine screening of the apparently healthy has no place in medical care as repeated studies have shown that while the so called risk factors can all be controlled with drugs and other interventions, the real risk, if any, of precocious death, remains unaltered!

The largest multiple risk factor intervention trial (MRFIT), followed for 25 long years at a phenomenal cost to the American Tax payer, made it loud and clear the message of futility of screening efforts save the added death and disability caused by adverse drug reactions, which incidentally happens to be one of the leading causes of death in the world.

Now let us glance at the recent conference conclusions:

* "With very few exceptions, the early screening and intervention touted by preventive medicine has turned out to be an oversold, dangerous, and expensive flop.

* Routine PSA screening for prostate cancer is the clearest example. It used to be recommended that men of a certain age be tested yearly. It is now recommended that the test not be done at all unless a man has a family history or other special risk factors.

* Definitive long term studies prove that the test doesn't save lives and instead ruins them by triggering invasive interventions with painful complications. Screening is usually too late to stop fast spreading tumours and too good at identifying slow growing ones that don't count and are better left alone.

If they live long enough, the majority of men will develop an incidental and benign prostate cancer before they die from something else. Picking up these tumours early causes great grief for no return.

* Lowering the thresholds of disease definitions has identified diseases that don't exist. The dream was that getting there early would help prevent the development of severe heart problems, hypertension, diabetes, osteoporosis, and a score of other illnesses.

The reality is that getting there too early misidentifies too many people who are not really at risk and then subjects them to needles and harmful tests and treatments.

* The technology is out of hand. If we do enough CT scans we can find structural abnormalities in just about everyone. But most findings are incidental and don't have any real clinical meaning. Paradoxically, lots of otherwise healthy people will get dangerous cancers from the CT radiation that served no useful purpose.

* Doctors have gotten into the habit of ordering huge batteries of laboratory tests and treating the results while ignoring what is best for this particular patient. There needs to be retraining of those already in practice, a change in how medicine is taught to new doctors, and a realignment of financial incentives to promote best care, not excessive care.

* Except for hospital care, it has become almost impossible to die in a dignified, humane, and cost effective way. Hospitals have become frenetic torture chambers that make dying much worse than death and cost an obscene fortune.

* Curing medical excess will not be easy. Harmful over testing and over treating is promoted and protected by the enormous economic and

political power of the medical industrial complex. Here's just a beginning list of what needs to be done.

* Tame and shame Big Pharma. Prohibit all Pharma contributions to professional associations and consumer groups. Regulate and make transparent all the marketing ploys used to mislead doctors. Force the publication of all clinical research trial data.

* Recognize that all existing medical guidelines that define disease thresholds and make treatment recommendations are suspect. They have been developed by experts in each field who always have an intellectual conflict of interest (and often enough also have a financial conflict of interest) that biases them toward over–diagnosis and overtreatment in their pet area of research interest. New diagnostic standards are as dangerous as new drugs and need the same careful and independent vetting to tame unrealistic diagnostic enthusiasm.

* Employers, insurance companies, and government payers should be smarter consumers of health services and should stop paying for tests and treatments that do more harm than good and are not cost effective.

* Consumers should be smarter consumers and not buy into the idea that more is always better.

* Medical journals need to be moiré skeptical of the medical research enterprise and should look toward the harms, not just the potentials, of each new purported advance. They should stop drum beating each new study as if it is another big step toward the cure for cancer which has proven more elusive than anyone imagined.

* The media needs to expose the real harms, not just the imagined wonders, inherent in medical procedures.

* We need to prove more resources to treat the really sick who now often get very inadequate care and at the same time need to protect the really well from getting what is often excessive and harmful care. It is wonderful that medical knowledge and tools have advanced so far, but disheartening that we are so bad at distributing them rationally.

* A great deal of progress has already been made. Fifty medical professional associations in the US have seen the need to cut back on inappropriate testing and treatment. Their `Choosing Wisely' initiative is a terrific start in reforming the disaster of our medical non system. The British Medical Journal and Consumers' Reports have already played a catalytic role and are powerful platforms for spreading the evidence to physicians and patients".

Now I am sure the western slavish mentality among our own colleagues will make them sit up and take note as this message has come from the west.

There were people from 28 countries in this conference in Hanover, although the problem of over diagnosis and over treatment is acute in the USA. India is catching up very fast and will soon over take USA as there are no official audits of treatment outcomes in India unlike the IOM audits in the USA. That worries me a lot.

That was the reason why I was belling the cat for the last four decades starting with my article in 1967 on :Should we be drugging every marginally elevated blood pressure? This, of course brought me lots of troubles. Coming from the western sources the above message (repeated verbatim in this write up) should have an impact.

"It was a lie but he believed in telling lies to people
Truth telling and medicine just didn't go together
except in dire emergencies, if then."

-Mario Puzo, The Godfather

THE REALITY STRIKES

THE ORDEAL ON THE MACHINE

Winter days were these, somewhere in January. She was counting the minutes or the hours? Lying down she would ask every ten minutes or so, how long ? We would keep telling her the minutes…The three hour ordeal, painful as it was would leave her totally drained out each time more than the previous. Her legs becoming thinner, face becoming smaller,shoulders looking so small, we saw her withering away,being sacrificed on the giant machine ,almost a monster. Once a person fell prey to it, there was no escape and none ever came back.,atleast I never saw one.

The poor old lady,now like a child, eagerly awaited the taxi, chiding that at last, it was over, and at least for a week she could be comfortable.

Her fluid intake was going on being decreased by the doctor. Whatever she adjusted to, was withdrawn. No lassi, no Coke, no Pepsi, no Limca………… nariyal pani?.....no, not even that. Water? ….limited.

The limit went on being decreased… My Billy would pine for some cold drink, some nariyal pani, but even water, it was not to be. 17 tablets/capsules in the whole day and hardly 1/5 of a jug of water. This is what! This is what can be called a treatment?

She was slipping from our hands, quite fast. The machine was being used more frequently, the gaps being reduced, the duration being increased.

"Mummy, don't worry, we shall again go to Shimla and I shall pack your clothes in your new suit case."

"Are pehle ye dilux (dialysis) to theek ho lene de."

As if it was a common cold she was suffering.

It was difficult not to cry out, at the height of her innocence.

The overpowering smell of water, all over, in the dialysis section, gave a sinking feeling upon entering. My eyes would search her out in the row of patients, and then would shine the most glowing smile on this earth. Come pain, come torture, but she would be giving that unforgettable smile welcoming me back from my court, and ask me about things in court.

While in the ICU, she would make sure I had reserved and secured a place for myself in the lobby for the night.

THE ILLUSIVE BOTTLE

That evening I reached along with a friend and she seemed thrilled at something, and pointed out to a bottle lying close by, which was containing the excess fluid tapped out from her body that afternoon, and as a result of which she was feeling very fresh, comfortable and she was bubbling with joy, taking it, as if she stood cured of the problem.

"Look, this was the root cause of all my discomfort and now I am perfect" .

She had just woken up smiling, and looked like a little rabbit. My hopes also brightened and I smiled with joy too..

The relief was not to last for long. She was travelling fast, to meet the destiny. Only childlike that she was, she did not know. Nor could I accept.

The hospital was my home for the said about one and half month, for wherever she was, could be my home. I found tricks to find my way to the ICU from here or there, on this pretext or that. While touching her feet, I was moving out when she called me to ask where was the grain? (the grain that I used to get touched by her and then give to the cows)

In the morning, one day, while I was going, she called me and told a dream she had seen i.e we all were to go on a trip on train, but that when the train came, all of us boarded it, but when she was to step onto it, the train had moved, and left her behind. She could not board the train.

She also saw a dream of eating her favourite food i.e aaloo poori, boondi raita sooji halwa. I asked my second mother to prepare it. She did all that was desired and brought the entire meal to the hospital. These days mother had been shifted to a room. Poor lady, when the delicious food came before her, she was not able to have any thing, except one small bite. There was no appetite. The entire tiffin lay untouched.

Sitting in that room 3404 ,by her side, she was fast asleep. I was again drifting into those good times which had been just until recently.

THE RECALL

We both were going to dharamshala by my omni. We had got late. In fact I had lost the route and by the time we reached Kiratpur it was already almost 6 pm. Going by this it was clear that we would not be there until midnight. I had laid a mattress for her in the back seat for her to be comfortable. But the tireless lady did not lie down for long and sat up. I asked her to take dinner at a café on way but she wouldn't. "Hotel pahunch kar khayenge''. Poor thing she was not realizing that we had miles and miles to go. Finally we reached around 1.30 am and obviously there were no chances of food. I managed to get milk and some kurkure was already with us. Scolding her like a kid "I told you so'' and all that. She munched on those kurkure and looked so cute.

Oh! Wish that day could come back, we were free in the fresh mountain air, she was perfectly enjoying the trip, the twinkle in her eyes, as the van would go around the turns and she was full of awe, saying every now and then "Are how do you manage to remember all these inter winding roads," and I would just smile it off gleefully, all the way.

Deep into the forests, on the river banks, in the rain, in the winter sun, she would be next to me sitting cozy and snuggled, chuckling away with her mango slice? She would often question me "look, where is the disease? I m perfectly fine. Who says I am not well or I have any problem?"

Even I used to do the routine check up through the BP machine and the glucometer. Even to my own surprise, the readings came in ranges whenever we were away from the city of Delhi and the house. Throughout in the hills, she remained perfect.

Gradually in routine check ups got done by the doctor sister, one or the other parameters were not as they should be and medicines multiplied one after another. After her bypass surgery, things were put in control of a nurse day long till I was in court.

My mom was made to feel she was seriously ill when she was not. Even if the problem was there the solutions were not in sight, except increase of medicine, reduction of water intake and then these machines.

BEYOND MY REACH

No one even believed in alternative therapy and cure. My running pillar to post was no use now. Dosages were heavy, in fact, she was beyond my reach now, as a patient. I kept doing my best ,I would keep giving her homeopathic medicine brought as per advice, but in the face of 17 tablets and capsules and the machines, what that dose could do.

I was called to the ICU and was told by the doctor, that she would have to be put on a ventilator. Not aware about the implications, I enquired and was told, that yes there is pain, as a pipe would be inserted in her throat, and thereafter also, she may, or may not, come out of it. In other words, she may spend the rest of her days on that not able to eat, not able to talk, just a vegetable existence.! For my mother? My bubbling little kitten ,my tavel partner ? No, Never, Never!

Doctors were now showing helplessness, just within six months of this hateful and painful process of Hoemo Dialysis.

It was the night. Around 9.30 the doctor called me and my sister to tell us with surprise that mom was responding to the homeopathic medicine perhaps and the congestion of fluid in her lungs was breaking up.

She was coughing and that was supposed to be a good sign.

Respite from our agony ,we were relieved and after many days, we had a proper meal in the café in the hospital complex. We, i.e my sister and myself were even laughing, relieved of our stressful moments. I had found the secret passage to the ICU, where I could sneak in, as and when, without any pass or permission and go and see her, always glowing, charming face, and could touch her holy feet.

THE YELLOW - FLIP FLOPS

Oh she had grabbed the chapels of Flight which I had brought for myself. Yellow and navy blue as light as a feather. She loved them, and they were hers; for good.

A week before in the room 3404, Sunday morning, she stopped responding and nervously we both called the doctor. Back to the ICU ,this time an ICU of the coronary department which somehow unusually had a fair share of sunlight streaming therein, her face shined, but still no movement. Doctor on duty was attending, but inspite of everything, she would not respond. I then asked her if she would like her, favourite drink of iced tea ?

And lo! She woke up, her eyes wide open! And nodded her head in a Yes. I rushed and ran, and tumbled and got her the ice tea. She got up, consumed the entire glass on her own with no help required, she smiled her cute kitten like smile and looked so fresh. She then told me, she was fine, and she would now sleep comfortably.

She slept on her side, curled up like a child and relieved, I started to leave the ICU. Duty doctor was amazed at the change.

THE FINAL CALL

26th May 2006, the bed was 2121, I had left her there and was in my sleeping bag in the lobby of first floor along with my sister. Around midnight, we were called in, and she was told to be in trouble. The pipes and paraphernalia were all in place, and my Billy was passing difficult moments. My hanuman chalisa, maha mrityunjoy path were all incessant. Now she was better and was recognizing every one, including me. We were told to leave.

27th May 2006, Saturday, 7.30 AM, Sleep had got the better of me, and I was cozily snuggled in my bag. "Attendants of Mrs Vimla Kohli (my billi), Please come to the ICU" the words announced on the mike, was the last announcement for us. But I had not known this. I rushed in my eagerness, that I would get a bonus visit to the ICU today, in addition, to the permitted ones.

Once inside, it was as if the world was slipping away like sand out of my hands. The doctors, nurses, all were surrounding her and trying to do something which I later came to realize, was to resuscitate her. I could not make out any thing. The doctor indicated to the nurse silently something and she started removing all the tubes and pipes away from my mother. Still I did not understand what had happened. Such a fool I was, I thought she had got better and did not require the tubes.

Then he indicated to me that I could meet her. I stepped forward with my usual excitement. But then I saw. Her head had rolled down to one side. The machine showing her heart rate, pulse rate was showing a flat straight line.

Everything was gone. The whole world was gone from me. My Billy was no more. My travel partner, my friend was no more. No one else mattered any more. For me no one was there any more. Finished. My pride had gone. My life, my joy had gone. World came to an end and nothing existed any more.

AWAY FROM GLITTER

They were doing a process and they gave me some daily use articles of my mother, like the 'flip flops' she had liked a lot, besides other articles.

They made her ready to leave with us. She was rolled down the stretcher and wheeled through another lift, in fact which had been the secret passage discovered by me, just a day before to meet her. We reached the basement, to a portion of the hospital, away from the glittering lights of the lobby, and the café and hub of the hospital . We were waiting for the Hearsay van.

The papers were being prepared. Around 8.45 am I was handed over the papers, and my mom. The van had arrived for the journey home.

She had left home on 19th April for just a routine check up but was detained never to return.

One of those days at the step down ICU, we were allowed to feed her. She didn't feel like having the breakfast but was being compelled to. She wanted water, just water, and that was being forbidden. What kind of treatment was it I could never make out. The nurse would come, and just wet her lips with a dripping cotton ball.

The van had reached home. Then she looked so beautiful even in death, I was yet to see a lady of her age so full of grace and the face so full of life. Among the usual ceremonies, started her last journey from home.

My life turned upside down. 'Maawan thandian chhawan…..' (mothers lap is like the shade of huge tree) the famous lines got understood by me.

The soul of the house was gone only the structure remained.

THE RETURN

Around 1 or 2 am in the midnight ,it was perhaps the third day, She came, looked at all of us for checking our well being, and reassured , she left.

The windscreen of my van used to get shower of water droplets many times, even though there was no visible source. She was meeting me in my dreams each passing night and I felt she was with me, and had not left me. She had not died. She was so alive.

One year had passed, and my feeling of suffocation had increased .I was restless and not just knowing what I could do now. That was the night she came to see me, not in her usual attire and looking pleasant. She told me that if I continued to cry like this, she would come only in this form ,but that if I smiled and remained happy, She would come to meet me in my dream every night.

That was the last day when I must have cried for her. I was assured she was fine over there, and infact better ! Out of the hell called ICU !

EPILOGUE

It was nine years later, I could never visualize myself, face to face, once again, with the monstrous machine, meant for carrying heamo dialysis.

This time it was my sister.... who was to be sacrificed on the machine... day by day... hour by hour.... minute by minute ...I saw her withering away ... dying down.... met the same agony, torture..... but all with the smile of innocence. In the hope that it was temporary and that one day perhaps, she would recover......

Once again our so-called medical science had no answer. No cures, no treatment... only increase in medicines, increase in problems, decrease in chances of survival.... experiments conducted upon her, one or another.

Worse was to come... the machine called `ventilator' the beginning of complete darkness... her helpless eyes... beseeching upon us to get everything removed... we laymen in the dark confused, in a dilemma.. I still see her reaching out to me... almost begging, to get all these gadgets and paraphernalia removed, her speech gone .... her voice lost.... one more life lost….. one more bond broken …. another departure from the ICU.

Was this a place to treat people ? What kind of treatment…. a step, by step push towards the end… is what it is !

I look at the birds flying…. parallel to the mountain tops… perhaps my mother is there in the clouds above….awaiting to receive her… with open arms.

Life goes on …. and yet, with the questions looming large in the mind……about the innocent believing millions of ailing people, thronging the corridors of the OPDs, occupying the beds in the ICUs, the mechanical and callous manner in which they are treated; and the heartless monstrous machines ….. how long shall all this continue ? ?

AND THE SONG ECHOES

Today I am just left singing to myself, on a winding mountain road, all by myself, the famous lines of this song, trying to reach out to my Mother…….

Chalo Chale Ma

Chalo Chale Ma Sapana Ke Ganv Me Kanto Se Dur Kahin Phulo Kee Chhanv Me

Chalo Chale Ma

Ho Rahe Ishare Reshamee Ghatao Me

Chalo Chale Ma

Aao Chale Ham Ek Sath Vaha

Dukh Na Jahan Koyee Gam Na Jahan

Aaj Hai Nimantran San Sani Havao Me

Chalo Chale Maa, Sapana Ke Ganv Me

Kanto Se Dur Kahin Phulo Kee Chhanv Me

Chalo Chale Ma

Rahana Mere Sang Ma Har Dam

Aisa Na Ho Ke Bichhad Jaye Ham

Rahana Mere Sang Ma Har Dam

Aisa Na Ho Ke Bichhad Jaye Ham

Ghumana Hai Hamko, Dur Ki Dishao Me

Chalo Chale Maa, Sapano Ke Ganv Me

Kanto Se Dur Kahin Phulo Kee Chhanv Me

Chalo Chale Ma

***